American Medical Association

Physicians dedicated to the health of America

State Medical Licensure Requirements and Statistics

2000-2001

AMA press

State Medical Licensure
Requirements and Statistics

©2000 by the American Medical Association
All rights reserved
Printed in the United States of America

Internet address: www.ama-assn.org

Additional copies of this book may be ordered by calling 800-621-8335.
Secure online orders can be taken at www.ama-assn.org/catalog.
Mention product number OP399000

Comments or inquiries
Fred Donini-Lenhoff, Editor
Medical Education Products
American Medical Association
515 North State Street
Chicago, IL 60610
312 464-5333
312 464-5830 Fax
E-mail: fred_lenhoff@ama-assn.org
www.ama-assn.org/licensure

ISBN 1-57947-064-5
BP15/0156-00

Foreword

State Medical Licensure Requirements and Statistics 2000-2001 presents current information and statistics on medical licensure in the United States and possessions. Data were obtained from a number of sources, including state boards of medical examiners, the Federation of State Medical Boards, National Board of Medical Examiners, Educational Commission for Foreign Medical Graduates, and the United States Medical Licensing Examination Secretariat.

Licensure data and policies in this publication were compiled from the AMA's 2000 Medical Licensure Survey, which was sent in April 2000 to all 54 allopathic boards of medical examiners in the United States. Although every effort was made to collect and record accurate data for each board, users of this book should note that the boards meet frequently and, as a result, their licensure and examination policies are modified regularly. It is therefore recommended that the state licensing boards (see Appendix A) be contacted for the most up-to-date information.

New in This Edition

A new table, "State Medical Board Standards for Administration of the USMLE, Steps 1 and 2," has been added to this year's edition. In addition, data on licensure for retired physicians is now available in Table 15.

Due to the difficulty in obtaining accurate data, the state-by-state licensure statistics that appeared in Section II of previous editions have been deleted. In the future, as improved procedures for collecting and verifying these data are developed, they will be available on the AMA's new Medical Licensure Online Web site at www.ama-assn.org/licensure.

Acknowledgments

The editors would like to thank the personnel of the state licensing agencies who provided statistics and licensing requirements for this publication. Acknowledgments are also due to the following individuals and organizations for their assistance with updating copy and writing articles:

- American Board of Medical Specialties—Stephen H. Miller, MD, MPH, Executive Vice President
- Robert D. Aronson, Esquire
- Department of the Air Force—Gary H. Murray, Brigadier General, USAF, DC, Commander, Air Force Medical Operations Agency; Sharon R. Ahrari, Lieutenant Colonel, USAF, NC, Deputy Chief, Clinical Performance Improvement, Office of the Surgeon General
- Department of the Army—Sid W. Atkinson, MD, Colonel, Director, Quality Management, US Army Medical Command
- Department of the Navy—Georgi Irvine, Commander, Nurse Corps, US Navy; John Chandler, Commander, Medical Corps, US Navy
- Drug Enforcement Administration, Office of Diversion Control—Patricia M. Good, Chief, Liaison and Policy Section
- Educational Commission for Foreign Medical Graduates—Stephen S. Seeling, JD, Vice President for Operations; Liz Ingraham, Project Coordinator
- Federation of State Medical Boards of the United States—Patricia Beatty, Assistant Vice President
- National Board of Medical Examiners—Kathleen T. Herron, Assistant Director, Department of Administration
- United States Medical Licensing Examination Secretariat—Kenneth E. Cotton

The editors would also like to acknowledge the contributions of the following AMA staff: Suzanne Fraker, Reg Schmidt, Jean Roberts, Anne Serrano, and Ronnie Summers of AMA Press; Enza Messineo and Hannah Hedrick, PhD, of Medical Education Products; and Arthur Osteen, PhD, Greg Paulos, and Julie Johnston of the Continuing Physician Professional Development.

Fred Donini-Lenhoff, Editor

Barbara S. Schneidman, MD, MPH, Director, Division of Medical Education Liaison and Outreach

Contents

List of Tables and Appendixes

Section I.

Licensure Policies and Regulations of State Medical Boards

State Medical Board Standards for Administration of the United States Medical Licensing Examination Step 3

In 1990, the Federation of State Medical Boards (FSMB) and the National Board of Medical Examiners (NBME) established the United States Medical Licensing Examination (USMLE), a single examination for assessment of US and international medical school students or graduates seeking initial licensure by US licensing jurisdictions. The USMLE replaced the Federation Licensing Examination (FLEX) and the certification examination of the NBME, as well as the Foreign Medical Graduate Examination in the Medical Sciences (FMGEMS), which was formerly used by the Educational Commission for Foreign Medical Graduates (ECFMG) for certification purposes.

The USMLE is a single examination program with three steps. Each step is complementary to the others; no step can stand alone in the assessment of readiness for medical licensure. Each USMLE step is composed of multiple-choice questions, requires 2 days of testing, and is administered semiannually. Additional information on the USMLE appears on p. 54.

Many states require US or Canadian medical school graduates to have from 6 months to 1 year of accredited US or Canadian graduate medical education (GME) to take USMLE Step 3. Graduates of foreign medical schools are generally required to have completed more GME (as much as 3 years in several states). A number of states do not require completion of GME to take Step 3 or require only that a physician taking the examination be enrolled in a GME program.

Nearly all medical licensing authorities require completion of Steps 1, 2, and 3 within a 7-year period (exceptions are Rhode Island, which requires passage within 6 years; California and Kansas, which allow 10 years; and Idaho, Louisiana, Michigan, New York, and North Carolina, which do not impose a time limit). This 7-year period begins when the medical student or graduate first passes Step 1 or Step 2. Many licensing authorities also limit the number of attempts allowed to pass each step.

Additional Notes for Specific Licensing Jurisdictions

Maryland—Seven-year to pass all 3 Steps of USMLE extended to 10 years for those in MD/PhD or similar programs.

Michigan—An applicant who fails to achieve a passing score on USMLE Step 3 within 5 years from the first attempt will not be eligible to again sit for USMLE Step 3 until completion of 1 year of GME in a board-approved program in the state.

Texas—Note A: Applicants for licensure must pass each part of the USMLE within three attempts, but an applicant who has passed all but one part within three attempts may take the remaining part of the examination one additional time.

Notwithstanding the above, an applicant is considered to have satisfied the requirements if the applicant 1) passed all but one part of a board-approved examination within three attempts and passed the remaining part within five attempts; 2) is specialty board certified by an ABMS or AOA specialty board; and 3) completed an additional 2 years of board-approved GME in Texas.

Note B: An extension of the 7-year period for completing all three steps of the USMLE will be allowed for applicants who pursue a simultaneous MD/PhD or DO/PhD program. This extension will not exceed the second anniversary of the date the MD or DO degree was awarded.

Virgin Islands—The USMLE is not administered; SPEX is used to evaluate physicians' knowledge.

Washington—Individuals completing a dual profession program, in which the applicant has met the required 1 year of GME outside the 7 years from passing the first examination, are allowed an additional 3 years for the three attempts following completion of GME.

Table 1
State Medical Board Standards for Administration of the US Medical Licensing Examination Step 3

	Amount of Accredited US or Canadian Graduate Medical Education Required to Take USMLE Step 3		Number of Times Candidates for Licensure May Take USMLE Step 3	Amount of Time Within Which All Steps of USMLE Must Be Passed
	Graduates of US/Canadian Medical Schools	Graduates of Foreign Medical Schools		
Alabama	10 mos	2 yrs, 10 months	4	7 yrs
Alaska	1 yr	1 yr	1	7 yrs
Arizona	6 mos	6 mos	No limit	7 yrs
Arkansas	1 yr	1 yr	6	7 yrs
California	None	None	No limit	10 yrs
Colorado	1 yr	1 yr	No limit	7 yrs
Connecticut	None	None	No limit	7 yrs
Delaware	1 yr	1 yr	3	7 yrs
DC	1 yr	3 yrs	No limit	7 yrs
Florida	1 yr	2 yrs	5	7 yrs
Georgia	1 yr	1-3 yrs	3	7 yrs
Guam	Not applicable	Not applicable	Not applicable	Not applicable
Hawaii	None (must be enrolled in 1st yr of GME prgm)	None (must be enrolled in 2nd year of GME prgm)	No limit	7 yrs
Idaho	9 mos	2 yrs, 9 mos	2 (after 2 failed attempts, remedial training required)	No limit
Illinois	1 yr	1 yr	5	7 yrs
Indiana	6 mos	2 yrs (if passed ECFMG exam pre-7/84, 3 yrs GME required)	3	7 yrs
Iowa	7 mos	7 mos	2	7 yrs
Kansas	1 yr	2 yrs	3 (after 3 failed attempts, further education, training, or experience required to repeat exam)	10 yrs
Kentucky	1 yr	1 yr	No limit	7 yrs
Louisiana	None	None	4	No limit
Maine	1 yr	1 yr (plus ECFMG certificate)	3	7 yrs
Maryland	None	None	No limit	7 yrs
Massachusetts	1 yr	1 yr	6	7 yrs
Michigan	6 mos	6 mos	No limit (after 5 yrs, further training required to repeat exam)	No limit
Minnesota	None (but must be enrolled in GME prgm)	None (but must be enrolled in GME prgm)	3	7 yrs
Mississippi	1 yr	3 yrs	3	7 yrs
Missouri	1 yr	3 yrs	3	7 yrs
Montana	1 yr	3 yrs	3	7 yrs
Nebraska	None	None	4	7 yrs
Nevada	1 yr	1 yr	No limit	7 yrs
New Hampshire	1 yr	1 yr	3 (after 3 failed attempts, further education, training, or experience required to repeat exam)	7 yrs (if not passed, must repeat entire sequence)

Table 1 (continued)
State Medical Board Standards for Administration of the US Medical Licensing Examination Step 3

| | Amount of Accredited US or Canadian Graduate Medical Education Required to Take USMLE Step 3 | | Number of Times Candidates for Licensure May Take USMLE | Amount of Time Within Which All Steps of USMLE Must Be Passed |
	Graduates of US/Canadian Medical Schools	Graduates of Foreign Medical Schools		
New Jersey	1 yr	1 yr	5 (after 5 failed attempts, further education, training, or experience required to repeat exam)	7 yrs (if not passed, must repeat entire sequence)
New Mexico	1 yr	1 yr	6	7 yrs
New York	None	None	No limit	No limit
North Carolina	None	3 yrs	No limit	No limit
North Dakota	1 yr	1 yr	4	7 yrs
Ohio	1 yr	1 yr	No limit	7 yrs
Oklahoma	10 mos	10 mos	3 (after 3 failed attempts, on any part, specialty board certification required)	7 yrs
Oregon	1 yr	1 yr	No limit	7 yrs
Pennsylvania	None (but must be enrolled in GME prgm)	None (but must be enrolled in GME prgm)	No limit (after 3 failed attempts, further education required)	7 yrs
Puerto Rico	None	None	No limit	7 yrs
Rhode Island	1 yr	1 yr	4	6 yrs
South Carolina	1 yr	3 yrs	4	7 yrs
South Dakota	1 yr	1 yr	3	7 yrs
Tennessee	1 yr	1 yr	No limit	7 yrs
Texas	None	None	3 (see Note A)	7 yrs (see Note B)
Utah	None	none (must be ECFMG-certified)	3 (remedial training required after 3 failed attempts)	7 yrs
Vermont	1 yr	1 yr	2	7 yrs
Virgin Islands	Not applicable	Not applicable	Not applicable	Not applicable
Virginia	1 yr	3 yrs	3	7 yrs
Washington	9 mos	9 mos	3 (remedial training required after 3 failed attempts)	7 yrs
West Virginia	none	none	No limit	7 yrs
Wisconsin	1 yr	1 yr	3	7 yrs
Wyoming	1 yr	2 yrs	2	7 yrs

Abbreviations

USMLE—United States Medical Licensing Examination
ECFMG—Educational Commission for Foreign Medical Graduates
GME—graduate medical education

Note: *All information should be verified with the licensing board; medical licenses are granted to those physicians meeting all state requirements—at the discretion of the board.*

State Medical Board Standards for Administration of the United States Medical Licensing Examination Steps 1 and 2

In 1990, the Federation of State Medical Boards (FSMB) and the National Board of Medical Examiners (NBME) established the United States Medical Licensing Examination (USMLE), a single examination for assessment of US and international medical school students or graduates seeking initial licensure by US licensing jurisdictions. The USMLE replaced the Federation Licensing Examination (FLEX) and the certification examination of the NBME, as well as the Foreign Medical Graduate Examination in the Medical Sciences (FMGEMS), which was formerly used by the Educational Commission for Foreign Medical Graduates (ECFMG) for certification purposes.

The USMLE is a single examination program with three steps. Each step is complementary to the others; no step can stand alone in the assessment of readiness for medical licensure. Each USMLE step is composed of multiple-choice questions, requires 2 days of testing, and is administered semiannually. Additional information on the USMLE appears on page 54.

The majority of medical licensing authorities do not place any limits on the number of times a candidate for licensure may take USMLE Steps 1 or 2 or on the amount of time needed to complete both steps.

Additional Notes for Specific Licensing Jurisdictions

Texas—Note A: Applicants for licensure must pass each part of the USMLE within three attempts, but an applicant who has passed all but one part within three attempts may take the remaining part of the examination one additional time.

Notwithstanding the above, an applicant is considered to have satisfied the requirements if the applicant 1) passed all but one part of a board-approved examination within three attempts and passed the remaining part within five attempts; 2) is specialty board certified by an ABMS or AOA specialty board; and 3) completed an additional 2 years of board-approved GME in Texas.

Note B: An extension of the 7-year period for completing all three steps of the USMLE will be allowed for applicants who pursue a simultaneous MD/PhD or DO/PhD program. This extension will not exceed the second anniversary of the date the MD or DO degree was awarded.

Table 2
State Medical Board Standards for Administration of the US Medical Licensing Examination Steps 1 and 2

	Number of Times Candidates for Licensure May Take USMLE Step 1	Number of Times Candidates for Licensure May Take USMLE Step 2	Amount of Time Within Which Steps 1 and 2 of USMLE Must Be Passed
Alabama	No limit	No limit	No limit
Alaska	1	1	7 yrs
Arizona	No limit	No limit	No limit
Arkansas	6	6	7 yrs
California	No limit	No limit	10 yrs
Colorado	No limit	No limit	No limit
Connecticut	No limit	No limit	No limit
Delaware	No limit	No limit	No limit
DC	No limit	No limit	No limit
Florida	No limit	No limit	No limit
Georgia	No limit	No limit	No limit
Guam	Not applicable	Not applicable	Not applicable
Hawaii	No limit	No limit	No limit
Idaho	2	2	No limit
Illinois	5	5	7 yrs
Indiana	No limit	No limit	No limit
Iowa	2	2	No limit
Kansas	No limit	No limit	No limit
Kentucky	No limit	No limit	No limit
Louisiana	No limit	4	No limit
Maine	No limit	No limit	No limit
Maryland	No limit	No limit	No limit
Massachusetts	No limit	No limit	No limit
Michigan	No limit	No limit	No limit
Minnesota	3	3	No limit
Mississippi	No limit	No limit	No limit
Missouri	3	No limit	No limit
Montana	No limit	No limit	No limit
Nebraska	4	4	No limit
Nevada	No limit	No limit	7 yrs
New Hampshire	2	2	7 yrs
New Jersey	No limit	No limit	7 yrs
New Mexico	No limit	No limit	No limit
New York	No limit	No limit	No limit
North Carolina	No limit	No limit	No limit
North Dakota	4	4	7 yrs
Ohio	No limit	No limit	7 yrs
Oklahoma	3	3	No limit
Oregon	No limit	No limit	No limit

Table 2 (continued)
State Medical Board Standards for Administration of the US Medical Licensing Examination Steps 1 and 2

	Number of Times Candidates for Licensure May Take USMLE Step 1	Number of Times Candidates for Licensure May Take USMLE Step 2	Amount of Time Within Which Steps 1 and 2 of USMLE Must Be Passed
Pennsylvania	No limit	No limit	No limit
Puerto Rico	No limit	No limit	7 yrs
Rhode Island	1	1	6 yrs
South Carolina	4	4	7 yrs
South Dakota	3	3	No limit
Tennessee	No limit	No limit	No limit
Texas	3	3 (see Note A)	No limit (see Note B)
Utah	No limit	No limit	No limit
Vermont	No limit	No limit	7 yrs
Virgin Islands	Not applicable	Not applicable	Not applicable
Virginia	No limit	No limit	No limit
Washington	No limit	No limit	No limit
West Virginia	No limit	No limit	7 yrs
Wisconsin	No limit	No limit	No limit
Wyoming	No limit	No limit	No limit

Endorsement Policies of State Boards for Physicians Holding an Initial License

Policies of medical licensing boards for endorsements of medical licensing examinations taken before and after the development of the Federation Licensing Examination (FLEX) vary from state to state. Each state board created its own licensing examination before FLEX, which may partially explain the sizable variation in endorsement policies from one state to another. Some boards will endorse scores on state licensing examinations in use prior to the development of FLEX, which may be endorsed in connection with a passing score on the Special Purpose Examination (SPEX). Endorsement of a certificate of the National Board of Medical Examiners (NBME) or of an examination refers to issuance of a license based on an acceptable score on the NBME or the state's board exam.

Endorsement relates to the issuance of licenses to physicians who hold licenses in other states or jurisdictions. Each state has strict endorsement requirements.

Thirty-five state medical boards require some or all candidates for licensure endorsement to appear for an interview; five (Idaho, Maine, North Carolina, Wisconsin, and Wyoming) require some or all candidates to appear for an oral examination.

Fourteen boards require that a license be endorsed within a certain period after examination (usually 10 years, but 3 months in Delaware). In most of these 14 states, SPEX is required if the time limit is not met.

All medical boards will accept or consider for endorsement the national board certificate of the NBME or the United States Medical Licensing Examination (USMLE), except the Virgin Islands, which does not accept endorsements. Forty-four boards will endorse the Licentiate of the Medical Council of Canada (LMCC); 16 will endorse a state board examination (designated "SBE" in Table 3) from another jurisdiction, occasionally in combination with a certificate from an American Board of Medical Specialties (ABMS) specialty board; six will endorse an ABMS board certificate; and eight will endorse the certificates of the National Board of Osteopathic Medical Examiners (NBOME). (Endorsement of these credentials is subject to any specific requirements in effect in that state.)

Additional Notes for Specific Licensing Jurisdictions

Colorado, Mississippi—LMCC is accepted or considered for endorsement for graduates of US or Canadian medical schools only.

Delaware—A candidate who took FLEX more than three times before June 1985 will not be eligible for licensure by endorsement, unless the candidate completes 1 additional year of training acceptable to the board. In that case, SPEX will be required.

Idaho—FLEX scores obtained at different sittings cannot be combined. Applicants who fail to pass the FLEX or USMLE on two separate occasions will not be eligible to take the examination for at least 1 year, and before taking either examination again, they must show the board that they have successfully engaged in a course of study to improve their ability to engage in the practice of medicine.

Illinois—Applicant had to pass all three parts of the pre-1985 FLEX in the same state.

Louisiana, Minnesota, Mississippi, Oregon, Texas—SPEX may be waived if an applicant was certified or recertified by an ABMS board within 10 years of the application date; Minnesota also may waive the SPEX requirements if an applicant is certified by a Canadian specialty board.

Maryland—SPEX is required if active licensure was interrupted during the last 10 years and if physician has not passed a written licensure exam within the last 15 years and the ABMS certification exam within the last 10 years.

Mississippi—FLEX scores obtained at different sittings cannot be combined.

Texas—All candidates for licensure must appear, present original documents for inspection, and pass the Texas Medical Jurisprudence Examination.

Candidates who have not been examined for licensure in the preceding 10-year period prior to filing their application must pass the SPEX
-or- have passed a specialty certification/recertification examination or formal evaluation or an examination of continued demonstration of qualifications by an ABMS or Bureau of Osteopathic Specialist member board within the preceding 10 years
-or- have obtained, through extraordinary circumstances, unique training equal to the training required for specialty certification as determined by a committee of the board and approved by the board.

Table 3
Endorsement Policies of State Medical Boards for Physicians Holding an Initial License

	Requirements for Endorsement of License Based on the Federation Licensing Examination (FLEX)			Requirements for Candidates' Appearance			Maximum Time for Licensure Endorsement After Examination		Credential Also Accepted or Considered for Endorsement (in addition to USMLE and NBME)
	Exceptions to 75 FWA on 3-part FLEX	Must Pass 3-Part (pre-1985) FLEX in One Sitting	Must Pass 2-Part (1985-93) FLEX in One Sitting	Candidates Who Must Appear...	...for Oral Exam	...for Interview	Time	Additional Requirements if Time Limit Not Met	
Alabama	None	No	No	Some			10 yrs	SPEX, ABMS	LMCC
Alaska	None	No	No	Some		X	None		LMCC, NBOME
Arizona	None	Yes	No	Some		Some	10 yrs	SPEX, ABMS	LMCC
Arkansas	None	Yes	No	IMGs		X	None		LMCC
California	None	Yes	No	None			10 yrs	SPEX	LMCC
Colorado	None	Yes	No	None			None		LMCC
Connecticut	Pre-6/85: 75 on day 3 to combine best scores (within 7 yrs); FWA truncated	No	No	None			None		LMCC (2 years GME US or abroad)
Delaware	None	No	No	All		X	3 mos	Training, SPEX	LMCC
DC	None	Yes	No	None			None		LMCC
Florida	None	Yes	No	Some		X	None		
Georgia	None	Yes	No	Some		X	None		LMCC
Guam	None	Yes	Yes	All		X	None		ABMS
Hawaii	None	No	No	None			None		
Idaho	See note	Yes	No	Some	Some	Some	5 yrs	SPEX	LMCC, SBE, NBOME
Illinois	None	No	No	Some		X	None		LMCC, NBOME
Indiana	Split scores okay	No	No	Some		X	None		LMCC
Iowa	None	Yes	No	Some		X	None		LMCC, SBE
Kansas	No scrambled scores	Yes	No	Some		X	None		LMCC, SBE (pre-1972)
Kentucky	None	Yes	No	Some			None		LMCC, SBE (pre-1972)
Louisiana	None	Yes	No	Some		X	10 yrs	SPEX	SBE
Maine	None	No	No	All	X		None		LMCC, GMC
Maryland	None	Yes	No	None			15 yrs	SPEX	LMCC
Massachusetts	None	Yes	No	Some		X	None	Current evaluations	LMCC (with Canadian provincial license), ABMS
Michigan	None	Yes	No	None			None		LMCC, SBE
Minnesota	None	Yes (5 tries)	No (3 tries)	All		X	10 yrs	SPEX, ABMS	LMCC, NBOME, SBE
Mississippi	See note	Yes	No	All		X	10 yrs	SPEX, ABMS	LMCC, NBOME
Missouri	None	Yes	No	Some		X	None		LMCC
Montana	None	Yes	No	Some		X	None		LMCC

Table 3 (continued)
Endorsement Policies of State Medical Boards for Physicians Holding an Initial License

	Requirements for Endorsement of License Based on the Federation Licensing Examination (FLEX)			Requirements for Candidates' Appearance			Maximum Time for Licensure Endorsement After Examination		Credential Also Accepted or Considered for Endorsement (in addition to USMLE and NBME)
	Exceptions to 75 FWA on 3-part FLEX	Must Pass 3-Part (pre-1985) FLEX in One Sitting	Must Pass 2-Part (1985-92) FLEX in One Sitting	Candidates Who Must Appear...	...for Oral Exam	...for Interview	Time	Additional Requirements if Time Limit Not Met	
Nebraska	None	Yes	No	None			None		LMCC, SBE
Nevada	None	No	No	Some		X	10 yrs	SPEX	ABMS (w/i 10 yrs of primary certification)
New Hampshire	None	No	No	None			None	May require exam, interview, proof of clinical competence, etc	LMCC, SBE
New Jersey	Pre-1/81: 74.5 FWA	No	No	Some		X	None		ABMS with license in another state, LMCC plus ABMS and license in another state
New Mexico	None	No	No	All		X	None		LMCC, SBE (pre-1970)
New York	None	No; 5-year period to pass all parts	No; 5-year period to pass all parts	None			None		LMCC (with a valid Canadian provincial license), ABMS, foreign license
North Carolina	1980-85: Day 1=70, Days 2 and 3=75	Yes	No	All	Some	X	10 yrs	Training, SPEX, AMA PRA	SBE, ABMS
North Dakota	None	Yes	No	Some		X (some)	None		SBE, LMCC, NBOME
Ohio	72 if taken during first 2 yrs of a state's administration and accepted as passing by state	Yes	No	None			None		LMCC (professional experience in US or abroad)
Oklahoma	None	Yes	No	Some		X	None		LMCC
Oregon	None	Yes	No	Some		X (some)	7 yrs	SPEX	LMCC
Pennsylvania	None	Yes	No	None			None		LMCC
Puerto Rico	None	Yes	Yes	None			None		
Rhode Island	None	No	No	Some		X	None		LMCC, NBOME
South Carolina	Pre-6/85: 75 FWA with no daily score below 70	Yes	No	All		X	10 yrs	SPEX	SBE with ABMS
South Dakota	None	Yes	Yes	Some		X	None		LMCC
Tennessee	None	Yes	Yes	Some		X	None		LMCC, ABMS
Texas	None	Yes	No	All		X	10 yrs	SPEX	LMCC, NBOME, COMLEX
Utah	None	No	No	Some		X	None		LMCC, SBE
Vermont	None	Yes	Yes (passed within 1 yr)	All		X	None		LMCC, ABMS

Table 3 (continued)
Endorsement Policies of State Medical Boards for Physicians Holding an Initial License

	Requirements for Endorsement of License Based on the Federation Licensing Examination (FLEX)			Requirements for Candidates' Appearance			Maximum Time for Licensure Endorsement After Examination		Credential Also Accepted or Considered for Endorsement (in addition to USMLE and NBME)
	Exceptions to 75 FWA on 3-part FLEX	Must Pass 3-Part (pre-1985) FLEX in One Sitting	Must Pass 2-Part (1985-92) FLEX in One Sitting	Candidates Who Must Appear...	...for Oral Exam	...for Interview	Time	Additional Requirements if Time Limit Not Met	
Virgin Islands	No reciprocity or endorsement; All licensure candidates must sit for complete SPEX exam.								
Virginia	None	No (unless taken before 6/76)	Yes	Some		X	None		LMCC, pre-1970=SBE, post-1969=SBE with ABMS
Washington	None	No	No	None			None		LMCC (post-1969)
West Virginia	None	Yes	No	All		X	None		LMCC, SBE
Wisconsin	None	Yes	No	Some	X		None		LMCC (post-1978)
Wyoming	None	Yes	No	All	X	X	None		LMCC

Abbreviations

FWA—Federation Licensing Examination (FLEX) Weighted Average, which applied to the pre-1985 three-part FLEX and gave greater weight to parts 2 and 3; all states currently require a minimum passing score of 75 on each component of the post-1985 two-part FLEX.

ABMS—certification from a member board of the American Board of Medical Specialties

FLEX—Federation Licensing Examination

GMC—General Medical Council of England and Ireland

IMG—International medical graduate

LMCC—certification by the Licentiate of the Medical Council of Canada

NBME—certificate of the National Board of Medical Examiners

NBOME—certificate from the National Board of Osteopathic Medical Examiners

SBE—state board examination

SPEX—Special Purpose Examination

USMLE—United States Medical Licensing Examination

Note: *All information should be verified with the licensing board; licenses based on endorsement are granted to those physicians meeting all state requirements.*

Additional Requirements for Endorsement of Licenses Held by International Medical Graduates

In all states, international medical graduates (IMGs) seeking licensure by endorsement must meet the same requirements as US graduates (listed in Table 3), in addition to the requirements in Table 4.

All states except Oklahoma require that IMGs seeking licensure endorsement hold a certificate from the Educational Commission for Foreign Medical Graduates (ECFMG). In lieu of holding that certificate, a candidate for licensure in Kentucky and North Dakota may have passed a certification examination of an American Board of Medical Specialties (ABMS) board or, in Wisconsin, the Foreign Medical Graduate Examination in the Medical Sciences (FMGEMS).

About half of the boards require IMG candidates to have graduated from a state-approved foreign medical school; some also require 3 years of US or Canadian GME. A majority of jurisdictions also may require an interview or oral examination prior to endorsement.

Additional Notes for Specific Licensing Jurisdictions

California—Four years' licensure required for IMGs, in addition to 2 years of GME (or 1 year of GME plus ABMS or 1 year of GME plus SPEX).

Florida—Rules on clinical clerkships for IMGs adopted by the Florida Board before October 1986 do not apply to any graduate who had already completed a clinical clerkship or who had begun a clinical clerkship, as long as the clerkship was completed within 3 years.

Rhode Island—Candidate must have obtained supervised clinical training in the US as part of the medical school curriculum in a hospital affiliated with an LCME-accredited medical school or an ACGME-accredited residency.

Illinois—Candidate must have completed a 6-year postsecondary course of study, comprising 2 academic years of liberal arts instruction, 2 academic years in basic sciences, and 2 academic years in clinical sciences, while enrolled in the medical school that confirmed the degree.

Iowa—Requirement for graduation from a state-approved medical school is waived if candidate passed the Special Purpose Examination (SPEX) or state science examination, or completed 3 years of GME in an ACGME-accredited residency program, or held a permanent license to practice without restrictions in a US jurisdiction for at least 5 years.

Maryland—As of October 1, 2000, 2 years of ACGME- or American Osteopathic Association-accredited GME required.

Michigan—Candidate must have completed specific basic science courses and clinical clerkships in hospitals approved by the state board.

Minnesota—SPEX is required if candidate took initial licensing exam more than 10 years ago, unless candidate is ABMS or Canadian medical specialty board-certified.

New Jersey—The ECFMG certificate requirement is waived for holders of the Fifth Pathway.

North Dakota—The ECFMG certificate requirement is waived for holders of the Fifth Pathway and for graduates of medical schools in Canada, England, Scotland, Ireland, Australia, or New Zealand. The requirement may be waived, by unanimous vote of the Board, for holders of ABMS certification.

The requirement for 3 years of US/Canadian GME is waived if the candidate holds an ABMS board certificate or has passed SPEX and (a) has successfully completed 1 year of state-approved GME in the US or Canada (or 3 years of GME in the United Kingdom), (b) has other professional experience and training equivalent to GME years 2 and 3, and (c) meets all other licensing requirements.

Pennsylvania—Candidate must have graduated from a medical school listed with the World Health Organization.

Texas—All IMG candidates for licensure must appear for interview, present original documents for inspection, and pass the Texas Medical Jurisprudence Examination.

West Virginia—The requirement for 3 years of GME in the US can be fulfilled with 1 year of GME in the US plus ABMS board certification.

Table 4
Additional Requirements for Endorsement of Licenses Held by International Medical Graduates
IMGs must also meet all the requirements for endorsement listed in Table 3

State	Candidate Must Have ECFMG Certificate	Candidate Must Have Graduated From a State-approved Foreign Medical School	Candidate Must Appear for... *(data summarized from Table 2)*
Alabama	Yes	Yes	SPEX (if no ABMS or SBE within 10 years)
Alaska	Yes	No	Possible interview
Arizona	Yes	No	SPEX if exam is over 10 yrs (and no current ABMS)
Arkansas	Yes	Yes	Interview
California	Yes	No	
Colorado	Yes	Yes	
Connecticut	Yes	Yes	
Delaware	Yes	No	Interview
DC	Yes	Yes	
Florida	Yes	No	Possible interview
Georgia	Yes	Yes	Possible interview
Guam	Yes	Yes	Possible interview
Hawaii	Yes	No	
Idaho	Yes	Yes	Possible oral exam; possible interview
Illinois	Yes	No	Possible interview
Indiana	Yes	No	Possible interview
Iowa	Yes	Yes	Possible interview
Kansas	Yes	No	Possible interview
Kentucky	Yes (or pass ABMS)	Yes	
Louisiana	Yes	Yes (3 years of GME in US also required)	Interview
Maine	Yes	No	Oral exam
Maryland	Yes	No	
Massachusetts	Yes	No	Possible interview
Michigan	Yes	No	
Minnesota	Yes	Yes (2 years of GME in US also required)	Interview, SPEX
Mississippi	Yes	Yes	Interview
Missouri	Yes	Yes	
Montana	Yes	Yes (3 years of GME in US also required)	Interview
Nebraska	Yes	No	
Nevada	Yes	No (3 years of GME in US or Canada required)	
New Hampshire	Yes	No	
New Jersey	Yes	No	Possible interview
New Mexico	Yes	Yes	Interview and orientation
New York	Yes	No	
North Carolina	Yes	No	Interview
North Dakota	Yes (or pass ABMS)	Yes (3 yrs GME in US/Canada also required)	Possible interview
Ohio	Yes	No	
Oklahoma	No	Yes	
Oregon	Yes	Yes (must be listed with WHO)	Possible interview
Pennsylvania	Yes	No (3 years of GME in US required)	
Puerto Rico	Yes	Yes	
Rhode Island	Yes	Yes (3 years of GME in US also required)	Possible interview
South Carolina	Yes	No (3 years of GME in US required)	Interview

Table 4 (continued)
Additional Requirements for Endorsement of Licenses Held by International Medical Graduates
IMGs must also meet all the requirements for endorsement listed in Table 3

	Candidate Must Have ECFMG Certificate	Candidate Must Have Graduated From a State-approved Foreign Medical School	Candidate Must Appear for... *(data summarized from Table 2)*
South Dakota	Yes	Yes	Possible interview
Tennessee	Yes	Yes	Possible interview
Texas	Yes	No (3 years of GME in US required)	Interview
Utah	Yes	No	Possible interview
Vermont	Yes	No (3 years of GME in US required)	Interview
Virginia	Yes	No	Possible interview
Washington	Yes	No	
West Virginia	Yes	No (3 years of GME in US required)	Interview
Wisconsin	Yes (or FMGEMS)	No	Possible oral exam
Wyoming	Yes	Yes (must be listed with WHO)	Full board interview

Abbreviations

ABMS—American Board of Medical Specialties

ECFMG—Educational Commission for Foreign Medical Graduates

FMGEMS—Foreign Medical Graduate Examination in the Medical Sciences

IMG—international medical graduate

SBE—state board examination

SPEX—Special Purpose Examination

VQE—Visa Qualifying Examination

WHO—World Health Organization

Note: All information should be verified with the licensing board; licenses based on endorsement are granted to those physicians meeting all state requirements.

Policies of State Medical Boards About the Special Purpose Examination (SPEX)

The Special Purpose Examination (SPEX), a 1-day, computer-administered examination with approximately 420 multiple-choice questions, assesses knowledge required of all physicians, regardless of specialty. SPEX is used to assess physicians who have held a valid, unrestricted license in a US or Canadian jurisdiction who are:

a) required by the state medical board to demonstrate current medical knowledge,

b) seeking endorsement licensure some years beyond initial examination, or

c) seeking license reinstatement after a period of professional inactivity. Physicians holding a valid, unrestricted license may also apply for SPEX, independent of any request or approval from a medical licensing board.

For more information on SPEX, see p. 61.

Forty-eight jurisdictions use SPEX to assess current competence or if a candidate has not taken a written licensure exam or the American Board of Medical Specialties (ABMS) board certification examination within a specified number of years (usually 10). In 22 states, SPEX scores are valid for an unlimited length of time. Forty jurisdictions will accept SPEX scores from other licensing jurisdictions.

Six US jurisdictions do not have SPEX policies— Massachusetts, New Jersey, Puerto Rico, Rhode Island, South Dakota, and Vermont. Of these, however, Puerto Rico will accept SPEX scores from other jurisdictions for licensure endorsement.

Additional Notes for Specific Licensing Jurisdictions

California—Four years' licensure in another state is required for international medical graduates.

Florida—SPEX is offered only to candidates who have actively practiced medicine for at least 10 years after obtaining a valid license in a jurisdiction or a combination of jurisdictions in the United States or Canada and who meet Florida's licensure requirements.

Maryland—SPEX is required if active licensure was interrupted during the last 10 years and if a physician has not passed a written licensure examination within the last 15 years and an ABMS board certification examination within the last 10 years.

Minnesota—SPEX scores are valid for an unlimited time, within three attempts.

North Dakota—SPEX (or ABMS board certification) is required when candidate is being considered for the following exception: If candidate has not completed 3 years of GME but has met all other licensing requirements and has successfully completed 1 year of US or Canadian GME in a board-approved program, and if the board finds that candidate has other professional experience and training substantially equivalent to the second and third years of GME, then candidate may be eligible for licensure.

Texas—SPEX scores accepted from other licensing jurisdictions if candidate passed with a score of 75 or higher.

Table 5
Policies of State Medical Boards About the Special Purpose Examination

	SPEX May Be Required...	...for the Following Reasons	...to Assess Current Competence	...if Written Licensure Exam or ABMS Certification Exam Has Not Been Taken Within	SPEX Scores Valid for	SPEX Scores Accepted from Other Licensing Jurisdictions
Alabama	Yes	By board order	X	10 years	10 years	Yes
Alaska	Yes	To restore a retired license	X		No limit	Yes
Arizona	Yes	By board order	X	10 years	10 years	Yes
Arkansas	Yes	By board order	X			Yes
California	Yes		X	10 years	10 years	Yes
Colorado	Yes	By board order	X			Yes
Connecticut	Yes		X			Yes
Delaware	Yes		X		No limit	Yes
DC	Yes	By board order	X			No
Florida	Yes		X		4 years	Yes
Georgia	Yes	By board order	X			Yes
Guam	Yes	By board order	X			Yes
Hawaii	Yes	If physician took a state licensing exam			No limit	Yes
Idaho	Yes	By board order	X		No limit	Yes
Illinois	Yes	Restore license after disciplinary action; if not been practicing for several yrs	X	(if state board exam taken before 1968)		Yes
Indiana	Yes		X			Yes
Iowa	Yes	If not been practicing for several yrs	X		No limit	Yes
Kansas	Yes	By board order	X		No limit	Yes
Kentucky	Yes	By board order	X		No limit	No
Louisiana	Yes		X	10 years	10 years	Yes
Maine	Yes	If not been practicing for 2 yrs	X		No limit	No
Maryland	Yes			15 years	No limit	Yes
Massachusetts	No					No
Michigan	Yes	For those with clinical academic license				No
Minnesota	Yes	Restore license after disciplinary action	X	10 years	No limit	Yes
Mississippi	Yes	Restore license after disciplinary action	X	10 years	10 years	Yes
Missouri	Yes	Restore license after disciplinary action	X		No limit	Yes
Montana	Yes	If not been practicing or inactive Montana license for last 2 yrs	X	2 years	No limit	Yes
Nebraska	Yes		X			Yes
Nevada	Yes			10 years	10 years	Yes
New Hampshire	Yes	By board order				No
New Jersey	No					No
New Mexico	Yes	If not been practicing for several yrs	X		No limit	Yes
New York	Yes	Determined on individual basis	X	(if state board exam taken before 1968)	No limit	Yes
North Carolina	Yes		X	10 years	10 years	Yes
North Dakota	Yes	(see note on previous page)	X		No limit	Yes
Ohio	Yes	If not been practicing for 2 yrs	X		No limit	Yes

Table 5 (continued)
Policies of State Medical Boards About the Special Purpose Examination

	SPEX May Be Required...	...for the Following Reasons	...to Assess Current Competence	...if Written Licensure Exam or ABMS Certification Exam Has Not Been Taken Within	SPEX Scores Valid for	SPEX Scores Accepted from Other Licensing Jurisdictions
Oklahoma	Yes		X			Yes
Oregon	Yes	If not been practicing for 1 yr, or no training or ABMS cert. for 10 yrs	X	10 years (or if state board exam taken before 1968)	10 years	Yes
Pennsylvania	Yes		X			Yes
Puerto Rico	No					Yes
Rhode Island	No					No
South Carolina	Yes	Restore license after disciplinary action; if not been practicing for 2 yrs	X	10 years	10 years	No
South Dakota	No					No
Tennessee	Yes	Restore license after disciplinary action; if license retired > 5 yrs	X		No limit	Yes
Texas	Yes		X	10 years	10 years	Yes
Utah	Yes	If not been practicing for several yrs; restore license after discipline	X			Yes
Vermont	No					No
Virgin Islands	Yes	To obtain licensure	X		No limit	No
Virginia	Yes		X		No limit	No
Washington	Yes	Restore license after disciplinary action; if not been practicing for 4 yrs	X		No limit	Yes
West Virginia	Yes		X		No limit	Yes
Wisconsin	Yes	Restore license after disciplinary action	X		No limit	No
Wyoming	Yes		X			Yes

Abbreviations

ABMS—American Board of Medical Specialties

SPEX—Special Purpose Examination

Note: *All information should be verified with the licensing board; medical licenses are granted to those physicians meeting all state requirements—at the discretion of the board.*

Policies of State Medical Boards
for Initial Medical Licensure
of US Medical School Graduates

All states require a written examination for initial licensure—generally the three-step United States Medical Licensing Examination (USMLE), which has replaced the Federation Licensing Examination (FLEX) and the national board examination of the National Board of Medical Examiners (NBME). For more information on the USMLE, see p. 54.

More than half of the state medical boards require graduates of US medical schools to have completed 1 year of graduate medical education (GME) to take USMLE Step 3. Fifteen boards do not require completion of any GME to take Step 3 (although in some cases a candidate must be enrolled in a GME program). All boards require completion of at least 1 year of GME before issuing a full, unrestricted license.

Table 6
Policies of State Medical Boards for Initial Licensure of US Medical School Graduates

	Amount of Accredited US or Canadian Graduate Medical Education Required	
	...to Take USMLE Step 3	...for Licensure
Alabama	10 mos	1 yr
Alaska	1 yr	2 yrs (1 yr if completed medical school before 1/95)
Arizona	6 mos	1 yr
Arkansas	1 yr	1 yr
California	None	1 yr
Colorado	None (must be enrolled in GME prgm)	1 yr
Connecticut	None	2 yrs
Delaware	1 yr	1 yr
DC	1 yr	1 yr
Florida	1 yr	1 yr
Georgia	1 yr	1 yr
Guam	1 yr	1 yr
Hawaii	None (must be enrolled in 1st year of GME prgm)	1 yr
Idaho	9 mos	1 yr
Illinois	1 yr	Entered GME pre-1/88, 1 yr; entered GME post-1/88, 2 yrs
Indiana	6 mos	1 yr (plus 1 yr GME if candidate failed any part of an exam 3 or more times and did not pass before 10/92)
Iowa	7 mos	1 yr
Kansas	1 yr	1 yr
Kentucky	1 yr	1 yr
Louisiana	None	1 yr
Maine	1 yr	2 yrs
Maryland	None	1 yr (plus 1 yr GME if candidate failed any part of an exam 3 or more times and did not pass before 10/92)
Massachusetts	1 yr	1 yr
Michigan	6 mos	2 yrs
Minnesota	None (must be enrolled in GME program)	1 yr
Mississippi	1 yr	1 yr
Missouri	1 yr	1 yr
Montana	1 yr	1 yr
Nebraska	None	1 yr
Nevada	1 yr	3 yrs
New Hampshire	1 yr	2 yrs
New Jersey	1 yr	1 yr
New Mexico	1 yr (must apply for public service license)	2 yrs
New York	None	1 yr
North Carolina	None	1 yr
North Dakota	1 yr (if not enrolled in in-state GME program; if enrolled in in-state program, can take at any time)	1 yr
Ohio	1 yr	1 yr
Oklahoma	10 mos	1 yr

Table 6 (continued)
Policies of State Medical Boards for Initial Licensure of US Medical School Graduates

	Amount of Accredited US or Canadian Graduate Medical Education Required	
	...to Take USMLE Step 3	...for Licensure
Oregon	1 yr	1 yr
Pennsylvania	None (must be enrolled in GME program)	2 yrs (1 yr if GME in US before 7/87)
Puerto Rico	None	1 yr
Rhode Island	1 yr	1 yr
South Carolina	1 yr	1 yr
South Dakota	1 yr	2 yrs (completion of residency)
Tennessee	1 yr	1 yr
Texas	None	1 yr
Utah	None	2 yrs
Vermont	1 yr	1 yr (Canadian GME accepted if program accredited by RCPSC
Virgin Islands	USMLE not offered	1 yr
Virginia	1 yr	1 yr
Washington	9 mos	2 yrs (1 yr if completed medical school before 7/28/85)
West Virginia	None	1 yr
Wisconsin	1 yr	1 yr
Wyoming	1 yr	1 yr

Abbreviations
USMLE—United States Medical Licensing Examination
GME—graduate medical education
RCPSC—Royal College of Physicians and Surgeons of Canada

Note: *All information should be verified with the licensing board; medical licenses are granted to those physicians meeting all state requirements—at the discretion of the board.*

Policies for Initial Medical Licensure of Canadian Citizens Who Are Graduates of Accredited Canadian Medical Schools

When considering applications for licensure, all state medical boards consider Canadian citizens who have graduated from an accredited Canadian medical school on the same basis as graduates of accredited US medical schools.

Forty-four licensing boards endorse the Licentiate of the Medical Council of Canada (LMCC) as evidence of passing an acceptable licensing examination (applicants must also pass all other board requirements for licensure).

With the exception of Guam, all medical boards accept Canadian graduation medical education (GME) as equivalent to GME in a US program accredited by the Accreditation Council for Graduate Medical Education (ACGME). These rules do not uniformly apply to international medical graduates, who should refer to Table 8.

Table 7
Policies of State Medical Boards for Initial Licensure of Canadian Citizens Who Are Graduates of Accredited Canadian Medical Schools

	Licentiate of the Medical Council of Canada (LMCC) Approved for Licensure by Endorsement	Graduate Medical Education in Accredited Canadian Programs Accepted as Equivalent to ACGME-accredited GME in the US	Notes
Alabama	Yes	Yes	
Alaska	Yes	Yes	
Arizona	Yes	Yes	
Arkansas	Yes	Yes	
California	Yes	Yes	
Colorado	Yes	Yes	
Connecticut	Yes	Yes	
Delaware	Yes	Yes	
DC	Yes	Yes	
Florida	No	Yes	
Georgia	Yes	Yes	
Guam	No	No	
Hawaii	No	Yes	
Idaho	Yes	Yes	
Illinois	Yes	Yes	Candidates who did not receive LMCC after 4/70 must be board certified or must complete USMLE Step 3 or the Special Purpose Examination
Indiana	Yes	Yes	
Iowa	Yes	Yes	LMCC must be endorsed by provincial licensing board
Kansas	Yes	Yes	
Kentucky	Yes	Yes	
Louisiana	No	Yes	
Maine	Yes	Yes	
Maryland	Yes	Yes	
Massachusetts	Yes	Yes	LMCC considered *only* if applicant has valid provincial license
Michigan	No	Yes	
Minnesota	Yes	Yes	
Mississippi	Yes	Yes	
Missouri	Yes	Yes	Only if medical school graduate of Canadian medical school
Montana	Yes	Yes	
Nebraska	Yes	Yes	
Nevada	Yes	Yes	
New Hampshire	Yes	Yes	
New Jersey	No	Yes	LMCC considered *only* if applicant is licensed in US jurisdiction
New Mexico	Yes	Yes	
New York	Yes	Yes	LMCC considered *only* if applicant has valid provincial license
North Carolina	No	Yes	
North Dakota	Yes	Yes	
Ohio	Yes	Yes	1 yr graduate medical education or its equivalent required
Oklahoma	Yes	Yes	
Oregon	Yes	Yes	
Pennsylvania	Yes	Yes	Must have received LMCC after 5/70 and in English
Puerto Rico	No	Yes	LMCC considered *only* if applicant is licensed in US jurisdiction
Rhode Island	Yes	Yes	
South Carolina	No	Yes	
South Dakota	Yes	Yes	
Tennessee	Yes	Yes	
Texas	Yes	Yes	
Utah	Yes	Yes	
Vermont	Yes	Yes	
Virgin Islands	No	Yes	At board discretion
Virginia	Yes	Yes	
Washington	Yes	Yes	Must have received LMCC after 12/69
West Virginia	Yes	Yes	Must have received LMCC after 12/77
Wisconsin	Yes	Yes	
Wyoming	Yes	Yes	

Policies of State Medical Boards for Initial Licensure of International Medical Graduates

All international medical graduates (IMGs) must hold a certificate from the Educational Commission for Foreign Medical Graduates (ECFMG) examination before taking Step 3 of the United States Medical Licensing Examination (USMLE). For IMGs seeking licensure, Oklahoma is the only state that does not require an ECFMG certificate. (For more information on the ECFMG certificate, see p. 66.)

Thirty-seven states will endorse for licensure the Licentiate of the Medical Council of Canada (LMCC) when held by an IMG.

Fourteen state boards allow IMGs to take USMLE Step 3 before they have had GME in a US or Canadian hospital. All states, however, require at least 1 year of GME for licensure, and 27 states require 3 years. Candidates are not awarded a license until they undertake the required GME in the United States and meet other board requirements (eg, an ECFMG certificate, personal interview, payment of fees).

Fifth Pathway

In 1971, the AMA established Fifth Pathway, a program for US citizens studying abroad at foreign medical schools. The program requires that participants have

1. Completed, in an accredited US college or university, undergraduate premedical work of a quality acceptable for matriculation in an accredited US medical school;

2. Studied medicine in a foreign medical school listed in the WHO *World Directory of Medical Schools*; and

3. Completed all formal requirements of the foreign medical school except internship and/or social service. (Those who have completed all the requirements of the foreign medical school are not eligible.)

If the aforementioned criteria are met, the candidate may substitute the Fifth Pathway program for internship and/or social service in the foreign country. After receiving a Fifth Pathway certificate from an accredited US medical school, these US citizens are eligible to enter the first year of GME in the United States.

In 48 states, individuals who hold Fifth Pathway certificates (but not the ECFMG certificate) are eligible for licensure. Fifth Pathway certificate holders must pass Steps 1 and 2 of the USMLE before entering a GME program accredited by the Accreditation Council for Graduate Medical Education (ACGME).

Additional Notes for Specific Licensing Jurisdictions

California—If licensed in another state for 4 or more years, the physician must have 2 years of GME or 1 year of GME plus ABMS or 1 year of GME plus SPEX.

Florida—ECFMG certificate required for licensure if candidate is not a graduate of a foreign medical school approved by the Florida Board of Medicine (none has yet been approved).

Louisiana—Fifth Pathway may be counted as 1 year of required GME.

Maine—GME taken in Canada or the British Isles (accredited by a national body deemed equivalent to ACGME) may be considered qualifying on an individual basis.

Maine, Wyoming—Oral examination is required for IMGs.

Maryland—As of October 1, 2000, 2 years of ACGME- or American Osteopathic Association-accredited GME required for all IMGs.

Mississippi—Three years of US or Canadian GME required for licensure; if a candidate has not completed 3 years of GME but 1) has met all other licensing requirements, 2) has completed at least 1 year of GME in a board-approved US or Canadian program, and 3) is ABMS board-certified, then the candidate may be deemed eligible for licensure, upon board approval.

Mississippi, South Carolina—ABMS board certification required for candidates who completed the Fifth Pathway.

North Carolina—IMG candidates for licensure must pass North Carolina board examination (USMLE or Federation Licensing Examination [FLEX]).

North Dakota—One year of accredited US or Canadian GME required to take USMLE Step 3 if not enrolled in North Dakota GME program; if enrolled in-state, candidate can take Step 3 at any time.

Three years of US or Canadian GME is required for licensure; if a candidate has not completed 3 years of GME but has met all other licensing requirements and has completed 1 year of GME in the United States or Canada in a board-approved program, and if the board finds that the candidate has other professional experience and training substantially equivalent to the second and third years of GME, the candidate may be deemed eligible for licensure (upon passing SPEX or ABMS board certification).

Oklahoma—An ECFMG certificate is not required for IMGs seeking licensure.

Oregon—IMG candidates for licensure must have completed at least 3 years of progressive GME in not more than two specialties in not more than two US or Canadian hospitals accredited for such training.

Pennsylvania—Board will grant unrestricted license by endorsement to a candidate who does not meet standard requirements if applicant has achieved cumulative qualifications that are endorsed by the board as being equivalent to the standard license requirements.

West Virginia—Fifth Pathway candidates must provide evidence of current ECFMG certification or a passing score on the ECFMG examination, along with successful completion of 3 years of GME in an ACGME-accredited program or 1 year of GME plus ABMS board certification.

Table 8
Policies of State Medical Boards for Initial Licensure of International Medical Graduates

	Accepts Physicians Who Complete a Fifth Pathway Program as Candidates for Licensure	Endorses Canadian Certificate (LMCC) Held by an IMG	Amount of Accredited US or Canadian Graduate Medical Education Required	
			...to Take USMLE Step 3	...for Licensure
Alabama	Yes	Yes	2 yrs, 10 mos	3 yrs
Alaska	No	Yes	1 yr	3 yrs
Arizona	Yes	Yes	6 mos	3 yrs
Arkansas	Yes	Yes	1 yr	1 yr
California	Yes	Yes	None	2 yrs (including 4 mos general med)
Colorado	Yes	Yes/No (case-by-case review)	None (must be enrolled in GME)	3 yrs
Connecticut	Yes	Yes	None	2 yrs
Delaware	Yes	No	1 yr	3 yrs
DC	Yes	Yes (oral exam may be required)	1 yr	1 yr
Florida	Yes	No	2 yrs	2 yrs
Georgia	Yes	No	1-3 yrs	3 yrs
Guam	No	No	1 yr	2 yrs (varies by specialty; Canadian GME not accepted)
Hawaii	Yes	No	None (but must be enrolled in 2nd year of GME program)	2 yrs
Idaho	Yes	No	2 yrs, 9 mos	3 yrs
Illinois	Yes	Yes	1 yr	1 yr (entered GME pre-1988); 2 yrs (entered GME post-1988)
Indiana	No	Yes	2 yrs	2 yrs
Iowa	Yes	Yes (with valid Canadian provincial license and fulfillment of all other licensure requirements)	7 mos	1 yr
Kansas	Yes	Yes	2 yrs	2 yrs
Kentucky	Yes	Yes	1 yr	3 yrs
Louisiana	Yes	No	None	3 yrs
Maine	Yes	Yes	1 yr (plus ECFMG certificate)	3 yrs
Maryland	Yes	Yes	None	2 yrs (as of 10/1/2000)
Massachusetts	Yes	Yes	1 yr	2 yrs
Michigan	No	No	6 mos	2 yrs
Minnesota	Yes	Yes	None (must be enrolled in GME)	2 yrs
Mississippi	Yes	No	3 yrs	3 yrs
Missouri	Yes	No	3 yrs	3 yrs
Montana	Yes	No	3 yrs	3 yrs
Nebraska	Yes	Yes	None	3 yrs
Nevada	Yes	Yes	1 yr	3 yrs
New Hampshire	Yes	Yes	1 yr	2 yrs
New Jersey	Yes	No	1 yr	3 yrs (1 yr if medical school completed before 7/1/85)
New Mexico	Yes	Yes	1 yr (must apply for public license)	2 yrs
New York	Yes	Yes (with valid Canadian provincial license and fulfillment of all other licensure requirements)	None	3 yrs

Table 8 (continued)
Policies of State Medical Boards for Initial Licensure of International Medical Graduates

	Accepts Physicians Who Complete a Fifth Pathway Program as Candidates for Licensure	Endorses Canadian Certificate (LMCC) Held by an IMG	Amount of Accredited US or Canadian Graduate Medical Education Required	
			...to Take USMLE Step 3	...for Licensure
North Carolina	Yes	No	3 yrs	3 yrs
North Dakota	Yes	Yes	1 yr	3 yrs
Ohio	Yes	Yes	1 yr	2 yrs (be enrolled in 2nd yr)
Oklahoma	Yes	Yes	10 mos	2 yrs
Oregon	Yes	Yes	1 yr	3 yrs
Pennsylvania	Yes	Yes (if passed after 5/70 and in English)	None (must be enrolled in GME program)	3 yrs (1 yr if GME taken in US before 7/87)
Puerto Rico	Yes	Yes	None	1 yr
Rhode Island	Yes	Yes (with valid Canadian provincial license and fulfillment of all other licensure requirements)	1 yr	1 yr
South Carolina	Yes	No	3 yrs	3 yrs
South Dakota	Yes	Yes	1 yr	2 yrs (1 yr if US GME taken before 7/87) and completion of residency
Tennessee	Yes	Yes	3 yrs	3 yrs
Texas	Yes	Yes	None	3 yrs
Utah	No	No	None	2 yrs
Vermont	No	No	1 yr	3 yrs (Canadian GME not accepted)
Virgin Islands	Yes	No	Not applicable	1 yr
Virginia	Yes	Yes	3 yrs (must be in 3rd yr)	3 yrs
Washington	Yes	Yes (if passed after 12/69)	9 mos	2 yrs (1 yr if medical school completed before 7/28/85)
West Virginia	Yes	Yes	None	3 yrs (or 1 yr plus ABMS certification)
Wisconsin	Yes	Yes (if passed after 12/77)	1 yr	1 yr
Wyoming	Yes	Yes	2 yrs	2 yrs

Abbreviations

GME—graduate medical education

IMG—International medical graduate

LMCC—Licentiate of the Medical Council of Canada

USMLE—United States Medical Licensing Examination

Note: All information should be verified with the licensing board; licenses are granted to those physicians meeting all state requirements—at the discretion of the board.

Medical Student Clerkship Regulations of State Medical Boards

For purposes of this publication, a clerkship is defined as clinical education provided to medical students. Twenty-two states evaluate the quality of clinical clerkships in connection with an application for licensure. In most states, clerkships for US medical students must take place in hospitals affiliated with medical schools accredited by the Liaison Committee on Medical Education (LCME). Twelve states have additional and/or more specific bases for evaluation.

Nineteen boards regulate clerkships provided in their states to students of foreign medical schools (including US citizens studying medicine in foreign schools). Of these, Pennsylvania, Puerto Rico, and Texas forbid such clerkships. For purposes of licensure, 19 states accept only those clerkships completed in hospital departments with graduate medical education (GME) programs accredited by the Accreditation Council for Graduate Medical Education (ACGME). Seven states have additional unspecified regulations.

Additional Notes for Specific Licensing Jurisdictions

California—Students of foreign medical schools may complete up to 18 of 72 required weeks in nonapproved clerkships outside of California.

Florida—Rules on clinical clerkships for international medical graduates adopted by the Florida Board before October 1986 do not apply to any graduate who had already completed a clinical clerkship or who had begun a clinical clerkship, as long as the clerkship was completed within 3 years.

An international medical school must be registered with the Florida Department of Education for its students to perform clinical clerkships in Florida.

Texas—Acceptance of clerkships in hospital departments with ACGME-accredited programs applies to those outside of Texas but within the US.

Table 9
Medical Student Clerkship Regulations of State Medical Boards

| State | Evaluates the Quality of Clinical Clerkships in Connection with a Licensure Application | Regulation of Clerkships Provided to Students of Foreign Medical Schools | | | |
		Regulates Clerkships Provided by Hospitals	Forbids Clerkships for Students of Foreign Med. Schools	Accepts Clerkships Only in Hospital Departments with ACGME-accredited Programs	Has Other Unspecified Regulations
Alabama	Yes	Yes		Yes	
Alaska					
Arizona					
Arkansas	Yes*	Yes		Yes	
California	Yes*	Yes		Yes	Yes
Colorado					
Connecticut	Yes*	Yes		Yes	
Delaware	Yes	Yes		Yes	
DC	Yes	Yes		Yes	
Florida	Yes	Yes		Yes	Yes
Georgia	Yes*	Yes		Yes	
Guam					
Hawaii					
Idaho					
Illinois	Yes	Yes		Yes	Yes
Indiana					
Iowa					
Kansas					
Kentucky	Yes	Yes		Yes	
Louisiana					
Maine	Yes			Yes	
Maryland					
Massachusetts	Yes*	Yes		Yes	Yes
Michigan					
Minnesota					
Mississippi					
Missouri					
Montana					
Nebraska					
Nevada					
New Hampshire					
New Jersey	Yes*	Yes		Yes	Yes
New Mexico	Yes*				
New York	Yes*	Yes		Yes	Yes
North Carolina	Yes*	Yes		Yes	
North Dakota					
Ohio					
Oklahoma					
Oregon	Yes	Yes		Yes	
Pennsylvania	Yes*	Yes	Yes	Yes	

Table 9 (continued)
Medical Student Clerkship Regulations of State Medical Boards

State	Evaluates the Quality of Clinical Clerkships in Connection with a Licensure Application	Regulation of Clerkships Provided to Students of Foreign Medical Schools			
		Adopted Regulations Governing Clerkships Provided by Hospitals	Forbids Clerkships for Students of Foreign Med. Schools	Accepts Clerkships Only in Hospital Departments with ACGME-accredited Programs	Has Other Unspecified Regulations
Puerto Rico	Yes	Yes	Yes		
Rhode Island	Yes				
South Carolina					
South Dakota					
Tennessee					
Texas	Yes*	Yes	Yes	Yes	Yes
Utah					
Vermont					
Virgin Islands					
Virginia	Yes*	Yes		Yes	
Washington					
West Virginia					
Wisconsin					
Wyoming					
Total	**22**	**19**	**3**	**19**	**7**

In many cases, clerkships must take place in hospitals affiliated with Liaison Committee for Medical Education (LCME)-accredited medical schools or Accreditation Council for Graduate Medical Education (ACGME)-accredited residency programs. States requiring additional and/or more specific criteria for evaluation are asterisked (*).

Note: All information should be verified with the licensing board; medical licenses are granted to those physicians meeting all state requirements—at the discretion of the board.

Additional Graduate Medical Education and Specialty Certificate Policies of State Medical Boards

A number of state medical boards have additional graduate medical education (GME) and specialty certificate policies for international medical graduates (IMGs). Fourteen states have requirements for appointment to GME programs other than requiring an Educational Commission for Foreign Medical Graduates (ECFMG) certificate or a limited license—Arizona, California, Connecticut, Iowa, Kansas, Kentucky, Louisiana, Michigan, Minnesota, Nevada, New Jersey, New Mexico, Pennsylvania, Texas, and Vermont.

Three boards—Connecticut, Maine, and Nebraska—indicated that GME completed in foreign countries other than Canada may be considered for credit toward a license. Specialty certificates of foreign boards, such as the Royal College of Physicians in the United Kingdom, are accepted for credit toward a license in nine states—Connecticut, Delaware, Maine, New York, Pennsylvania, Rhode Island, Tennessee, Utah, and Vermont.

Thirty-six medical boards accept GME accredited by the Accreditation Council for Graduate Medical Education (ACGME) for licensure of osteopathic medical graduates.

Additional Notes for Specific Licensing Jurisdictions

Maine—May accept GME completed in England, Scotland, and Ireland for credit toward a license.

May accept specialty certificates of boards in England, Scotland, and Ireland for credit towards a license, if accepted by specialty board as meeting board eligibility in the United States and notified via certified letter.

Pennsylvania—IMGs seeking appointment to a GME program need a passing score on United States Medical Licensing Examination (USMLE) Steps 1 and 2 (or National Board of Medical Examiners [NBME] Parts I and II or Federation Licensing Examination [FLEX] Component 1) for graduate year 2 medical education; for graduate year 3 and above, all parts of USMLE (or NBME or FLEX) are required.

Rhode Island—May accept specialty certificates of boards in England, Scotland, and Ireland for credit toward a license.

Table 10
Additional Graduate Medical Education and Specialty Certificate Policies of State Medical Boards

State	Has State Board Requirements for Appointment to GME Program Other Than ECFMG certificate or Limited License	May Accept GME Completed in Foreign Countries Other Than Canada for Credit Toward a License	May Accept Specialty Certificates of Foreign Boards (eg, Royal College of Physicians of the United Kingdom) for Credit Toward a License	Osteopathic Medical Graduates	
				ACGME-Accredited GME Accepted	State Osteopathic Board Handles Licensure
Alabama				Yes	
Alaska					
Arizona	Yes (residency permit required)				Yes
Arkansas				Yes	
California	Yes (must meet all undergraduate education requirements)				Yes
Colorado				Yes	
Connecticut	Yes (residency intern permit required)	Yes	Yes	Yes	
Delaware			Yes (case-by-case basis)	Yes	
DC					
Florida					Yes
Georgia					
Guam					
Hawaii					
Idaho				Yes	
Illinois				Yes	
Indiana				Yes	
Iowa	Yes (may require interview/exam)			Yes	
Kansas	Yes (unapproved school must have been in existence at least 15 yrs)			Yes	
Kentucky	Yes			Yes	
Louisiana	Yes (passage of FLEX/NBME/USMLE)			Yes	
Maine		Yes	Yes	Yes	Yes
Maryland				Yes	
Massachusetts				Yes	
Michigan	Yes (certification of medical education)				Yes
Minnesota	Yes (residency intern permit required)			Yes	
Mississippi				Yes	
Missouri				Yes	
Montana				Yes	
Nebraska		Yes		Yes	
Nevada	Yes (diploma, transcript)				Yes
New Hampshire				Yes	
New Jersey	Yes (residency intern permit required)			Yes	
New Mexico	Yes (residency intern permit required)				Yes
New York			Yes	Yes	
North Carolina				Yes	
North Dakota				Yes	
Ohio				Yes	

Table 10 (continued)
Additional Graduate Medical Education and Specialty Certificate Policies of State Medical Boards

	Has State Board Requirements for Appointment to GME Program Other Than ECFMG Certification or Limited License	May Accept GME Completed in Foreign Countries Other Than Canada for Credit Toward a License	May Accept Specialty Certificates of Foreign Boards (eg, Royal College of Physicians of the United Kingdom) for Credit Toward a License	Osteopathic Medical Graduates	
				ACGME-Accredited GME Accepted	State Osteopathic Board Handles Licensure
Oklahoma					Yes
Oregon				Yes	
Pennsylvania	Yes		Yes		Yes
Puerto Rico					
Rhode Island			Yes	Yes	
South Carolina				Yes	
South Dakota				Yes	
Tennessee			Yes; specialty board must be AMA-recognized		Yes
Texas	Yes (physician-in-training permit required)			Yes	
Utah			Yes	Yes	Yes
Vermont	Yes		Yes		Yes
Virgin Islands				Yes	
Virginia				Yes	
Washington					Yes
West Virginia					Yes
Wisconsin				Yes	
Wyoming				Yes	
Total	**15**	**3**	**9**	**36**	**14**

Abbreviations

ACGME—Accreditation Council for Graduate Medical Education
ECFMG—Educational Commission for Foreign Medical Graduates
FLEX—Federation Licensing Examination
GME—graduate medical education
NBME—certificate of the National Board of Medical Examiners
USMLE—United States Medical Licensing Examination

Note: *All information should be verified with the licensing board; medical licenses are granted to those physicians meeting all state requirements—at the discretion of the board.*

Accredited Subspecialties and Nonaccredited Fellowships That Satisfy GME Requirements for Licensure

Both the AMA and the Accreditation Council for Graduate Medical Education (ACGME) define a residency as graduate medical education (GME) that takes place in any of the more than 100 specialties or subspecialties that have ACGME Program Requirements (eg, the specialty of internal medicine, the subspecialty of cardiovascular disease). A fellowship is defined as clinical or research-oriented GME in an area of medicine that does not have ACGME Program Requirements.

All state medical boards accept residency education in specialty programs accredited by the ACGME as satisfying their GME requirements for licensure. Forty-nine jurisdictions—all except Arkansas, Guam, Montana, Pennsylvania, and Puerto Rico—accept residency education in subspecialty programs accredited by ACGME as satisfying their GME requirements for licensure.

Six boards accept clinical fellowships not accredited by ACGME, and three boards—Missouri, New York, and North Carolina—accept research fellowships not accredited by ACGME to satisfy the GME requirement for licensure.

Additional Notes for Specific Licensing Jurisdictions

Texas—Accepts clinical fellowships not accredited by ACGME if in Texas and board-approved.

Table 11
Accredited Subspecialties and Nonaccredited Fellowships That Satisfy Graduate Medical Education Requirements for Licensure

	Accepts Subspecialty GME Accredited by ACGME	Accepts Clinical Fellowships *Not* Accredited by ACGME	Accepts Research Fellowships *Not* Accredited by ACGME
Alabama	Yes (if clinical)		
Alaska	Yes		
Arizona	Yes		
Arkansas			
California	Yes		
Colorado	Yes		
Connecticut	Yes	Yes	
Delaware	Yes		
DC	Yes		
Florida	Yes		
Georgia	Yes		
Guam			
Hawaii	Yes		
Idaho	Yes		
Illinois	Yes		
Indiana	Yes		
Iowa	Yes		
Kansas	Yes		
Kentucky	Yes		
Louisiana	Yes		
Maine	Yes		
Maryland	Yes		
Massachusetts	Yes		
Michigan	Yes		
Minnesota	Yes		
Mississippi	Yes		
Missouri	Yes	Yes	Yes
Montana			
Nebraska	Yes		
Nevada	Yes	Yes	
New Hampshire	Yes		
New Jersey	Yes		
New Mexico	Yes		
New York	Yes	Yes	Yes
North Carolina	Yes	Yes	Yes
North Dakota	Yes		
Ohio	Yes		
Oklahoma	Yes		
Oregon	Yes		
Pennsylvania			
Puerto Rico			
Rhode Island	Yes		
South Carolina	Yes		
South Dakota	Yes		
Tennessee	Yes		
Texas	Yes	Yes	
Utah	Yes		
Vermont	Yes		
Virgin Islands	Yes		
Virginia	Yes		
Washington	Yes		
West Virginia	Yes		
Wisconsin	Yes		
Wyoming	Yes		
Total	**49**	**6**	**3**

Abbreviations

ACGME—Accreditation Council for Graduate Medical Education
GME—graduate medical education

**Note: *All information should be verified with licensing board;
medical licenses are granted to those physicians meeting all
state requirements—at the discretion of the board.***

Licensure Requirement Exemptions for Eminent Physicians and Medical School Faculty

Nine boards license physicians through recognition of eminence in medical education or medical practice. Physicians appointed to a medical school faculty are excused from the graduate medical education (GME) requirement for limited licensure in 15 states and from the examination requirement for limited licensure or teaching certification in 12 states. These faculty appointees would, however, receive a limited license or similar credential.

Additional Notes for Specific Licensing Jurisdictions

Colorado—Distinguished foreign physicians are invited to serve on faculty; temporary licensure may not exceed 2 years.

Florida, Iowa—Physicians appointed to a medical faculty are eligible for a special license, with which they may practice only at the designated facility/institution.

Georgia—Physicians appointed to a medical faculty are excused from the GME requirement for limited licensure for teaching only.

Louisiana—Physician licensed through recognition of eminence in medical education must be approved as a tenured professor/associate professor by a Louisiana medical school.

Montana—An international medical graduate (IMG) seeking a restricted license must have published in an English-language, peer-reviewed medical journal.

Ohio—Physicians appointed to a medical faculty are eligible for a visiting medical faculty certificate, with which they may practice only at the school or teaching hospitals affiliated with the school. This nonrenewable certificate is valid for 1 year or the duration of the appointment, whichever is shorter.

Texas—Physicians appointed as full medical school professors in a salaried full-time position may be designated Distinguished Professors and be excluded from the Special Purpose Examination (SPEX) if required under the 10-year rule.

Table 12
Licensure Requirement Exemptions for Eminent Physicians and Medical School Faculty

	License Physicians Through Recognition of Eminence in Medical Education or Practice	Physicians Appointed to a Medical Faculty Are Excused From...	
		...the Graduate Medical Education Requirement for Limited Licensure	...the Examination Requirement for Limited Licensure
Alabama			
Alaska			
Arizona		Yes	
Arkansas			
California	Yes	Yes	Yes
Colorado			
Connecticut		Yes	Yes
Delaware	Yes		
DC	Yes	Yes	Yes
Florida		Yes	Yes
Georgia		Yes (see note)	Yes
Guam			
Hawaii			
Idaho			
Illinois			
Indiana	Yes		
Iowa		Yes	Yes
Kansas			
Kentucky			
Louisiana	Yes	Yes	Yes
Maine			
Maryland	Yes	Yes	Yes
Massachusetts			
Michigan			
Minnesota			
Mississippi			
Missouri			
Montana	Yes		
Nebraska			
Nevada			
New Hampshire			
New Jersey			
New Mexico			
New York			
North Carolina	Yes	Yes	Yes
North Dakota			
Ohio		Yes	
Oklahoma			
Oregon			
Pennsylvania	Yes	Yes	
Puerto Rico			
Rhode Island		Yes	Yes
South Carolina			

Table 12 (continued)
Licensure Requirement Exemptions for Eminent Physicians and Medical School Faculty

	License Physicians Through Recognition of Eminence in Medical Education or Practice	Physicians Appointed to a Medical Faculty Are Excused From...	
		...the Graduate Medical Education Requirement for Limited Licensure	...the Examination Requirement for Limited Licensure
South Dakota			
Tennessee		Yes	Yes
Texas			
Utah			
Vermont		Yes	Yes
Virgin Islands			
Virginia			
Washington			
West Virginia			
Wisconsin			
Wyoming			
Total	**9**	**15**	**12**

Note: All information should be verified with the licensing board; medical licenses are granted to those physicians meeting all state requirements—at the discretion of the board.

Medical Licensure and Reregistration Fees and Intervals; CME Reporting Requirements

The National Board of Medical Examiners (NBME) administers United States Medical Licensing Examination (USMLE) Steps 1 and 2 to students and graduates of US and Canadian medical schools at test centers established by the NBME; application materials are usually available at these medical schools. The Educational Commission for Foreign Medical Graduates (ECFMG) administers USMLE Steps 1 and 2 to students and graduates of foreign medical schools; application materials are available only through the ECFMG.

Administration of USMLE Step 3 is the responsibility of the individual medical licensing jurisdictions. Step 3 application materials for physicians who have successfully completed Steps 1 and 2 are available from the medical licensing authorities or the Federation of State Medical Boards (FSMB), which administers the examination for 48 jurisdictions. (For more information on USMLE Step 3 in those states where it is administered by the FSMB, call 800 USMLE XM—800 876-5396). USMLE Step 3 fees, including *all examination costs and processing, application, and administrative fees*, range from $885 in Georgia to $225 in Virginia; the average is $501. (For additional information on USMLE, see p. 54.)

Fees for licensure by endorsement, *including processing, application, and administrative fees*, range from $1,108 in California to $20 in Pennsylvania; the average is $351.

The majority of boards require physicians licensed in the state to reregister (or renew) their licenses every 1 or 2 years; four jurisdictions—Illinois, Michigan, New Mexico, and Puerto Rico—have a 3-year reregistration interval. The reregistration fee ranges from $500 per year in the Virgin Islands to $15 per year in Indiana; the average reregistration fee is $153 per year. Many states offer reduced fees for reregistration of inactive licenses.

Completion and reporting of a specified number of hours of continuing medical education (CME) is required for reregistration in 37 jurisdictions.

Additional Notes for Specific Licensing Jurisdictions

Alaska—Reregistration fee is $100 for inactive license.

Arizona—If less than 10 years has elapsed since candidate passed a written examination for licensure in another state, endorsement fee is $550 (rather than $450), to include required Special Purpose Examination (SPEX).

Late penalty fee of $350 is charged if licensure reregistration is not submitted by February 1 of each year. License automatically expires on May 1 if renewal and late penalty fee are not submitted.

California—Endorsement fee includes $508 processing fee and $600 licensing fee. Resident physician applicants are charged a reduced fee of $300.

Colorado—Reregistration fee is $150 for inactive license.

Illinois—Reregistration fee for nonresidents is $600. Penalty of $100 is charged if renewal is not submitted by July 31 in the year of renewal.

Montana—Reregistration fee is $60 for inactive license.

Nevada—Reregistration fee is $200 for inactive license.

Oregon—Biennial inactive or out-of-state reregistration fee is $270 for inactive license.

Virginia—USMLE Step 3 examination fee is $85 without subsequent licensure or $225 with subsequent licensure.

Washington—Applicants for initial license endorsement must add a $25 fee.

West Virginia—Reregistration fee is $100 for inactive license.

Table 13
Medical Licensure and Reregistration Fees and Intervals; CME Reporting Requirements

State	Examination		Endorsement Fees	Licensure Reregistration		
	USMLE Step 3	Administered by FSMB		Registration Interval	Fee	CME Reporting Required
Alabama	$ 585		$ 175	1 yr	$ 100	Yes
Alaska	500	Yes	500	2 yrs	340	Yes
Arizona	450	Yes	450	1 yr	225	Yes
Arkansas	485	Yes	400	1 yr	70	Yes
California	485	Yes	1,108	2 yrs	600	Yes
Colorado	485	Yes	375	2 yrs	305	
Connecticut	485	Yes	450	1 yr	450	
Delaware	485	Yes	235	2 yrs	143	Yes
DC	655	Yes	300	2 yrs	120	
Florida	485	Yes	503	2 yrs	355	Yes
Georgia	885	Yes	400	2 yrs	150	Yes
Guam	355	Yes	400	2 yrs	250	Yes
Hawaii	485	Yes	290	2 yrs	240	Yes
Idaho	485	Yes	400	1 yr	200	
Illinois	400		300	3 yrs	300	Yes
Indiana	485	Yes	40	2 yrs	30	
Iowa	505	Yes	300	2 yrs	325	Yes
Kansas	420	Yes	250	1 yr	180	Yes
Kentucky	485	Yes	250	1 yr	125	Yes
Louisiana	485	Yes	200	1 yr	100	
Maine	485	Yes	400	2 yrs	400	Yes
Maryland	485	Yes	790 (890 for IMGs)	2 yrs	400	Yes
Massachusetts	450		350	2 yrs	250	Yes
Michigan	500	Yes	140	3 yrs	270	Yes
Minnesota	485	Yes	200	1 yr	192	Yes
Mississippi	500	Yes	500	1 yr	100	Yes
Missouri	450	Yes	450	1 yr	120	Yes
Montana	500	Yes	325	1 yr	200	
Nebraska	485	Yes	201	2 yrs	102	
Nevada	485	Yes	400	2 yrs	600	Yes
New Hampshire	485	Yes	250	1 yr	100	Yes
New Jersey	530	Yes	225	2 yrs	340	
New Mexico	485	Yes	350	3 yrs	310	Yes
New York	485		735	2 yrs	600	
North Carolina	755	Yes	250	1 yr	100	
North Dakota	485	Yes	200	1 yr	150	Yes
Ohio	400	Yes	335	2 yrs	305	Yes
Oklahoma	485	Yes	400	1 yr	150	Yes
Oregon	485	Yes	375	2 yrs	438	
Pennsylvania	485	Yes	20 (80 for IMGs)	2 yrs	125	
Puerto Rico	500		200	3 yrs	75	Yes
Rhode Island	485	Yes	350	1 yr	200	Yes
South Carolina	600	Yes	500	1 yr	80	Yes
South Dakota	605	Yes	200	1 yr	50	

Table 13 (continued)
Medical Licensure and Reregistration Fees and Intervals; CME Reporting Requirements

State	Examination		Endorsement Fees	Licensure Reregistration		
	USMLE Step 3	Administered by FSMB		Registration Interval	Fee	CME Reporting Required
Tennessee	485	Yes	235	2 yrs	110	
Texas	800	Yes	800	1 yr	330	Yes
Utah	485	Yes	150	2 yrs	100	Yes
Vermont	520	Yes	400	2 yrs	350	
Virgin Islands	No exam		Not applicable	1 yr	500	Yes
Virginia	85, 225	Yes	200	2 yrs	260	Yes
Washington	455	Yes	300	2 yrs	450	Yes
West Virginia	485	Yes	300	2 yrs	300	Yes
Wisconsin	485	Yes	96	2 yrs	110	Yes
Wyoming	485	Yes	350	1 yr	200	
Total/Average	**$501**	**48**	**$351**	**—**	**$153 (per year)**	**37**

Abbreviations

CME—continuing medical education

FSMB—Federation of State Medical Boards

IMG—international medical graduate

USMLE—United States Medical Licensing Examination

Note: *All information should be verified with the licensing board; medical licenses are granted to those physicians meeting all state requirements—at the discretion of the board.*

Continuing Medical Education for Licensure Reregistration

Thirty-seven boards require anywhere from 12 hours (Alabama) to 50 hours (several states) of continuing medical education (CME) per year for license reregistration. Some states also mandate CME content, such as HIV/AIDS, risk management, or medical ethics. Many states also require that a certain percentage of CME be category 1, as measured, for example, through the American Medical Association Physician's Recognition Award (for more information, see p. 90). In Ohio, all CME must be certified by the Ohio State Medical Association or the Ohio Osteopathic Association.

Additional Notes for Specific Licensing Jurisdictions

Maryland—Partial CME credit is offered for ABMS certification, select peer review, serving as a intervenor or monitor on a physician rehabilitation committee or professional committee, and serving as a preceptor for resident physicians or medical students in LCME-accredited schools.

Table 14
State Medical Board Regulations on Continuing Medical Education for Licensure Reregistration

State	Required Number of CME Hours per Year(s)		Average Hours per Year	AMA/AOA/AAFP/ACOG Category 1 Hours Required	Certificates Accepted as Equivalent*	State-mandated CME Content/ Additional Notes
Alabama	24	2 yrs	12	24	AMA, ACOG, AAFP	
Alaska	17	1 yr	17	17	AMA, ABMS, AOA, APA	
Arizona	20	1 yr	20		ABMS, GME	
Arkansas	20	1 yr	20	20		
California	100	4 yrs	25	100	AMA, AAFP, CMA, CAFP	
Colorado	none					
Connecticut	none					
Delaware	40	2 yrs	20	40	AMA, AOA	
DC	none					
Florida	40	2 yrs	20	40		HIV/AIDS, domestic violence, TB
Georgia	40	2 yrs	20	40		
Guam	100	2 yrs	50	25		
Hawaii	100	2 yrs	50	40	AMA	
Idaho	none					
Illinois	50	1 yr	50			
Indiana	none					
Iowa	40	2 yrs	20	40	AMA, AOA, GME	Child/dependent adult abuse
Kansas	150	3 yrs	50	60	AMA, ABMS, GME, AOA	
Kentucky	60	3 yrs	20	30		HIV/AIDS; course must be approved by Kentucky Cabinet for Hlth Svcs
Louisiana	none					
Maine	100	2 yrs	50	40	AMA, ABMS, AAFP	
Maryland	50	2 yrs	25	50		(see note)
Massachusetts	100	2 yrs	50	40	GME	Study board reqs; risk mgmt
Michigan	150	3 yrs	50	75	AMA	
Minnesota	75	3 yrs	25	75	AMA, AOA, MOCOMP	
Mississippi	40	2 yrs	20	40		
Missouri	25	1 yr	25		AAFP	
Montana	none					
Nebraska	none					
Nevada	40	2 yrs	20	40		ethics (2 hrs), 20 hrs in specialty
New Hampshire	150	3 yrs	50	60	AMA, ABMS	
New Jersey	none					
New Mexico	75	3 yrs	25	75	AMA, ABMS, AAFP, ACOG, USMLE	
New York	none					infection control, child abuse
North Carolina	none					
North Dakota	20	1 yr	20	20	AMA, AOA, AAFP, MOCOMP	
Ohio	100	2 yrs	50	40		Must be certified by OSMA or OOA
Oklahoma	150	3 yrs	50	60	AMA, board-recognized equivalent	
Oregon	none					
Pennsylvania	none					150 hrs of CME every 3 years required by state insurance agency
Puerto Rico	60	3 yrs	20	40		
Rhode Island	60	3 yrs	20	60		HIV universal precautions/ blood-borne pathogens
South Carolina	40	2 yrs	20	40	ABMS, AOA, ACOG equivalent	
South Dakota	none					
Tennessee	none					
Texas	24	1 yr	24	12		Of 12 hrs category 1, at least 1 hr in ethics/prof. responsibility
Utah	40	2 yrs	20	40		
Vermont	none					
Virgin Islands	40	1 yr	40	25		
Virginia	60	2 yrs	30	30		Of category 1, 15 hrs must be interactive
Washington	200	4 yrs	50		AMA, ABMS, AAFP, ACOG	
West Virginia	50	2 yrs	25	50	AMA, ABMS (partial)	
Wisconsin	30	2 yrs	15	30		
Wyoming	none					

ABMS—certification or recertification by a member board of the American Board of Medical Specialties; AMA—American Medical Association; AOA—American Osteopathic Association; AAFP—American Academy of Family Practice; ACOG—American College of Obstetricians and Gynecologists; APA—American Pediatric Association; CMA—California Medical Association; CAFP—California Academy of Family Physicians; CME—continuing medical education; FLEX—Federation Licensing Examination; GME—graduate medical education; MOCOMP—Royal College of Physicians and Surgeons of Canada; OSMA—Ohio State Medical Association; USMLE—United States Medical Licensing Association

Temporary or Limited Licenses, Permits, Certificates, and Registration Issued by State Medical Boards

Forty-five states issue educational licenses, permits, certificates, or registration to resident physicians in graduate medical education (GME) programs. (The GME program director generally provides a list of residents and any other required information directly to the licensing jurisdiction.) In 26 of those states, residents must obtain a new permit/license when changing residency programs within the state. In eight states—Arizona, California, Indiana, Kentucky, Massachusetts, Mississippi, New Hampshire, and New Mexico—prospective residents must have passed United States Medical Licensing Examination (USMLE) Step 1 to receive a permit/license. California requires passage of Steps 1 and 2.

Forty-six boards issue temporary and educational permits, limited and temporary licenses, or other certificates for the practice of medicine. The terms for the issuance of such certificates vary, but in general they must be renewed once a year with a stipulated maximum number of renewals allowed (usually 5 years).

Some states permit state institutions to hire unlicensed physicians to work under the supervision of licensed physicians. In many instances, the state departments of mental health and public health that operate these hospitals will not hire physicians who have not had at least 1 year of GME in an English-speaking hospital. International medical graduates are generally not considered for these positions unless they are in the United States with a permanent resident visa. An unlicensed physician employed by a state hospital is required in most states to register with the state board of medical examiners, which may issue a limited permit to practice within the institution.

Thirty-three states issue teaching (visiting professor) licenses, 15 issue locum tenens permits, and 25 issue inactive licenses (for physicians who want to maintain licensure in that state although they are currently practicing in another state). Eleven states offer a special licensure fee for retired physicians.

Table 15
Temporary or Limited Licenses, Permits, Certificates, and Registration Issued by State Medical Boards

	Residents and Prospective Residents			Temporary/Limited Licenses, Permits, and Certificates	Teaching (Visiting Professor) Licenses	Locum Tenens Permits	Inactive Licenses	Retired Physicians' Licenses
	Licenses, Permits, Certificates, & Registration	Must Obtain New Permit/License When Changing Residency Programs Within State	Prospective Residents Applying for License Must Have Passed USMLE Step 1					
Alabama				Yes	Yes			
Alaska	Yes			Yes		Yes	Yes	Yes
Arizona	Yes	Yes	Yes	Yes	Yes	Yes	Yes	
Arkansas				Yes				
California	Yes		Yes		Yes		Yes	Yes
Colorado					Yes		Yes	
Connecticut	Yes	Yes		Yes	Yes			
Delaware	Yes	Yes		Yes	Yes	Yes		
DC							Yes	
Florida	Yes	Yes		Yes	Yes		Yes	
Georgia				Yes	Yes		Yes	
Guam	Yes	Yes		Yes				
Hawaii	Yes			Yes	Yes			
Idaho	Yes			Yes			Yes	
Illinois	Yes	Yes		Yes	Yes		Yes	
Indiana	Yes	Yes	Yes	Yes	Yes	Yes	Yes	
Iowa	Yes	Yes		Yes	Yes		Yes	
Kansas	Yes			Yes	Yes		Yes	Yes
Kentucky	Yes		Yes	Yes				
Louisiana	Yes	Yes		Yes	Yes			Yes
Maine	Yes	Yes		Yes	Yes	Yes	Yes	
Maryland	Yes			Yes	Yes		Yes	
Massachusetts	Yes		Yes	Yes	Yes	Yes	Yes	
Michigan	Yes	Yes			Yes			
Minnesota	Yes	Yes		Yes				
Mississippi	Yes		Yes	Yes				Yes
Missouri	Yes	Yes		Yes	Yes			
Montana				Yes		Yes	Yes	
Nebraska	Yes	Yes			Yes	Yes	Yes	
Nevada	Yes	Yes		Yes		Yes	Yes	Yes
New Hampshire	Yes	Yes	Yes	Yes	Yes	Yes		
New Jersey	Yes	Yes		Yes				Yes
New Mexico	Yes		Yes	Yes	Yes			
New York	Yes			Yes				
North Carolina	Yes	Yes		Yes	Yes		Yes	
North Dakota	Yes			Yes		Yes		
Ohio	Yes	Yes		Yes	Yes		Yes	Yes
Oklahoma	Yes	Yes		Yes				Yes
Oregon	Yes	Yes		Yes	Yes			
Pennsylvania	Yes			Yes	Yes			Yes
Puerto Rico	Yes			Yes	Yes			
Rhode Island	Yes	Yes		Yes	Yes		Yes	
South Carolina	Yes	Yes		Yes				
South Dakota	Yes					Yes		
Tennessee	Yes	Yes		Yes	Yes	Yes	Yes	
Texas	Yes	Yes		Yes	Yes			
Utah	Yes						Yes	
Vermont	Yes				Yes			
Virgin Islands				Yes				
Virginia	Yes	Yes		Yes	Yes		Yes	Yes
Washington	Yes			Yes				
West Virginia				Yes		Yes	Yes	
Wisconsin	Yes			Yes	Yes	Yes		
Wyoming				Yes				
Total	**45**	**26**	**7**	**46**	**33**	**15**	**25**	**11**

Table 15 (continued)
Temporary or Limited Licenses, Permits, Certificates, and Registration Issued by State Medical Boards

Alabama
- Limited license for residency education and for work in state penal and mental institutions only.
- Teaching (visiting professor) licenses on a limited basis.

Alaska
- Temporary permits for specific period (6 months maximum) after completed application is on file and until board meets to consider permanent licensure.
- Locum tenens permit for 60 days to an MD or DO licensed in another state for purpose of substituting for another Alaska-licensed physician; may extend 3 times.
- Resident permits for up to 1 year to physicians in accredited residency programs in the United States.
- Retired physician license: $50 one-time fee

Arizona
- Locum tenens permit for a 180-day period to a licensed MD who must be sponsored by an Arizona-licensed physician, either MD or DO; issued only once in a 3-year period.
- Teaching licenses, for practice within the clinical training program only, to full-time faculty members teaching at an accredited medical school or residency/fellowship program.
- Education Training Permit, granted for 5 days

Arkansas
Temporary permits for limited time in emergency or hardship cases, only after application for licensure is complete and waiting to be presented to the board. Valid until next board meeting.

California
- Renewable certificates of registration (awarded on an individual basis) for 1-5 years to physicians who do not immediately meet licensure requirements and who have been offered full-time teaching positions in California medical schools.
- Permits (awarded on an individual basis) for maximum of 5 years to noncitizen physicians for postgraduate work in a California medical school.
- IMGs must submit an application to determine that all core requirements have been met.
- Biennially renewable faculty permit (awarded on an individual basis) issued to academically eminent physicians, for whom the medical school has assumed direct responsibility. The holder may practice medicine only within the sponsoring medical school and affiliated institutions.
- Retired physician license: Available at no charge

Connecticut
- Temporary permits (valid for 1 year only, not renewable or extendable) only to those physicians who have been offered a position in a state hospital or state facility.
- Resident/intern permits to individuals in accredited GME programs in Connecticut hospitals.

Delaware
- Temporary permit until board meets to approve candidates; locum tenens permit.
- Limited institutional license under supervision of licensed physician.

Florida
- Temporary Certificate to Practice in Area of Critical Need to MDs with current valid license in another state to practice in Florida communities with a critical need for physicians and a population of less than 7,500.
- Limited License to MDs who meet the same minimum education and training requirements as required for a full medical license and who are retired and have been licensed to practice medicine in any jurisdiction in the United States for at least 10 years. Practice restricted to public agencies or institutions or nonprofit agencies or institutions meeting the requirements of Section 501(c)(3) of the Internal Revenue Code and located in areas of critical medical need.
- A Public Psychiatry Certificate to board-certified psychiatrists who are licensed to practice medicine without restriction in another state and who meet the minimum education and training requirements required for a full medical license. Practice is restricted to a public mental health facility or program funded in part or entirely by state funds.
- A Public Health Certificate to MDs who are graduates of an accredited medical school and hold a master of public health degree or are board-eligible or certified in public health or preventive medicine, or to MDs who are licensed to practice medicine without restriction in another jurisdiction in the United States and hold a master of public health degree or are board eligible or certified in public health or preventive medicine and who meet the minimum education and training requirements required for a full medical license. Practice restricted to employment duties with the Department of Health and Rehabilitative Services.
- A Medical Faculty Certificate to MDs who are graduates of an accredited medical school or its equivalent and hold a valid current license to practice medicine in another US jurisdiction. Certificate authorizes practice only in conjunction with teaching duties at an accredited Florida medical school or in its main teaching hospitals. A 180-day permit; no more than three physicians per year per institution may hold this certificate; certificate can be granted to a physician only once in a given 5-year period.
- Registration of unlicensed physicians required.

Georgia
- Temporary permits for reciprocity/endorsement applicants between board meetings (fee $100).
- Teacher's license for faculty of approved Georgia medical schools (subject to terms and conditions).

Hawaii
- To physicians in accredited residency programs; to physicians working in a state or county agency in conditions of shortage or emergency; and to physicians under the supervision of a licensed MD who plan to take the USMLE exam within 18 months.
- Not available to physicians against whom disciplinary action is pending in another state.
- Teaching (Visiting Professor) licenses good for 1 year from date issued.

Idaho
Temporary license until next board meeting after application for licensure is complete; no requirements waived.

Table 15 (continued)
Temporary or Limited Licenses, Permits, Certificates, and Registration Issued by State Medical Boards

Illinois
- Temporary licenses (valid for not more than 3 years; may be extended or renewed) to persons in residency programs that are ACGME- or American Osteopathic Association-approved. License cannot extend beyond completion of the residency program.
- Limited temporary licenses (valid for 6 months) to persons in non-Illinois residency programs who are accepted for a specific period of time to perform a portion of that program at a clinical residency program in Illinois due to the lack of adequate facilities in their state.
- Visiting Professor Permits for 1 year (renewable once) to persons receiving faculty appointments to teach in either a medical or osteopathic school.
- Visiting Physician Permits for up to 180 days to persons receiving an invitation or appointment to study, demonstrate, or perform a specific medical, osteopathic, or chiropractic subject or technique in medical, osteopathic, or chiropractic schools; hospitals; or facilities operated pursuant to the Ambulatory Surgical Treatment Center Act.
- Visiting Resident Permits issued for 180 days to persons who have been invited or appointed for a specific period of time to perform a portion of that clinical residency program under the supervision of an Illinois-licensed physician in an Illinois patient care clinic or facility affiliated with the out-of-state graduate medical education program.

Indiana
- To physicians holding an active, valid license from another US/Canadian jurisdiction who have applied for and are awaiting board approval of permanent unrestricted license by endorsement of another jurisdiction's valid license; valid for a designated period of 90 days or less.
- To physicians holding a valid, active license from another US/Canadian jurisdiction who are providing health care for a circumscribed period as part of a special program, event, or other activity, including locum tenens; permit valid for up to 30 days and is not renewable.
- To an institution for a specific physician to whom it has granted a visiting faculty appointment. Requires that applying institution certify, to the satisfaction of the board, the qualifications of the physician. Practice of the physician limited to the applying institution for a designated period not to exceed 1 year.
- To physicians undertaking approved residency education in Indiana. Practice limited to the program/institution(s) of training for a period of 1 year; may be renewed annually.

Iowa
- Resident physician license for training in approved hospital under supervision of licensed physician.
- Temporary license at discretion of board for specific location, date, and need.

Kansas
- Temporary permit until next licensure board meeting after application for licensure has been completed, filed, processed, and found to be in order.
- Institutional permits to work in state institutions or mental health centers.
- Resident permit for residents, visiting clinical professor license, out-of-phase special permit.
- No temporary permit before passing examination.
- Physicians may request inactive status. Physicians with inactive licenses may not practice medicine in any form, including writing prescriptions.
- Retired physician license: $90 for inactive status

Kentucky
- Temporary permit until board meets (for endorsement candidates only).
- Institutional Practice Limited License to IMGs beyond first year of graduate medical education while in training.

Louisiana
- Unrestricted temporary permits only under extreme circumstances. Board meets every 6-8 weeks to act on reciprocity licensure applications. Board must act on SPEX applicants requiring unrestricted temporary permit. SPEX applicants issued institutional temporary permit, if necessary, pending results of exam.
- Intern registration for first 12 months of residency education after completing medical school.
- Ninety-day renewable unrestricted permit, pending valid visa issued by the Immigration and Naturalization Service.
- Retired physician license: $75

Maine
- Temporary seasonal camp licenses.
- Educational permits for 1 year in a specific training program, renewable for 5 years.
- Temporary (up to 1 year) for duration of community need.
- Licensees not meeting Maine's CME requirements are registered as inactive.

Maryland
- Registration of medical school graduates in graduate medical education programs
- Limited 1-year license for postgraduate teaching.
- Physicians may request inactive status. Physicians with inactive licenses may not practice medicine in any form, including writing prescriptions.

Massachusetts
- Limited registration for physicians enrolled in accredited residency programs and for physicians enrolled in fellowships at hospitals with accredited residency programs in the area of the applicant's specialty.
- Temporary registration for physicians who hold a temporary faculty appointment at a Massachusetts medical school, are substituting temporarily for a fully licensed Massachusetts physician, or are enrolled in a CME course that requires Massachusetts licensure. Physicians requesting temporary registration must be currently licensed in another state.

Michigan
Limited annual license (not to exceed 5 years) for graduate medical education, renewable each year.

Minnesota
Temporary license valid until next board meeting at which application is to be considered.

Mississippi
- Institutional license to interns and IMG physicians providing health care in state institutions. Applicants are *not* required to meet all requirements for permanent unrestricted licensure.
- Restricted temporary license to physicians enrolled in first year of graduate medical education at the University of Mississippi School of Medicine for practice limited to that school.
- Youth Camp Permit valid for 90 days issued to physicians for the provision of health care only at designated youth camps approved by the Mississippi State Department of Health.
- Addictionology Fellowship License to physicians admitted for treatment in a board-approved drug and/or alcohol addiction treatment program or to physicians enrolled in fellowship of addictionology of the Mississippi State Medical Association Impaired Professionals Program.

Table 15 (continued)
Temporary or Limited Licenses, Permits, Certificates, and Registration Issued by State Medical Boards

Missouri
- Issues temporary license only to interns, residents, and fellows.
- Retired physician license: $25 limited license

Montana
- Temporary license to physicians for practice in specified location in the interval between board meetings. Board may ask physician to appear at next board meeting for temporary license renewal. No requirements are waived.
- Thirty-day locum tenens permits available, but candidate must meet all requirements for licensure.

Nebraska
- Temporary educational permits for residents and temporary visiting faculty permits for medical school faculties.
- Locum tenens permit for a qualified physician with current license in another state for replacement of a Nebraska physician during a period of temporary leave (maximum of 90 days in any 12-month period).

Nevada
- Limited license for 1 year to residents in a clinical residency program.
- Locum tenens license (one-time only) for 3 months to qualified candidates.
- Temporary licenses for practice in medically underserved areas (at discretion of the board).
- Retired physician license: $50 every 2 years

New Hampshire
Temporary/restricted license, in the state's best interest. Locum tenens (courtesy license) available to a qualified applicant currently holding an unrestricted active license in another state; valid for a maximum of 100 days in any 12-month period.

New Jersey
- Temporary license (4 months) for a lawfully qualified physician of another state to take charge of the practice of a licensed New Jersey physician during his or her absence from the state. Exemption from licensure to work in county or state institution for a limited period.
- Retired physician license: $125

New Mexico
- Requires licensure of all resident physicians.
- Interim licenses until subsequent board meeting.
- Temporary camp licenses.
- Temporary licenses for out-of-state physicians (visiting professors) under sponsorship of New Mexico-licensed physician and teaching institution and mini-residencies.
- Physicians may request inactive status. Physician with an inactive license may not practice medicine in any form, including writing prescriptions.

New York
- Requires limited permit for all medical school graduates except individuals in ACGME- or AOA-accredited residency programs.
- Requires ECFMG certificate from all IMGs before issuing limited permit.

North Carolina
- Limited license to physicians in residency programs who are not eligible for licensure by endorsement.
- Limited license for practice in geographic areas with underserved populations
- Temporary licenses to eligible endorsement candidates beginning practice prior to board meeting.
- Limited faculty license for medical school faculty.

North Dakota
- Temporary license between intervals of board meetings, because an interview is required before a permanent license is issued. All licensure requirements must be met and file must be processed completely before a temporary license or locum tenens permit will be issued.
- Locum tenens permit, not to exceed 3 months.
- Limited license (1 year) for residents in a clinical program.

Ohio
- Training certificate or full license mandatory for participation in an accredited internship, residency, or clinical fellowship program
- Limited certificates for employment in state hospitals.
- Visiting Medical Faculty certificate and Special Activities certificates.
- Retired physician license: $100 for Emeritus certificate or Volunteer's certificate

Oklahoma
- Temporary medical licenses during the intervals between board meetings. Candidates for temporary license must meet qualifications for full and unrestricted license. Temporary licenses automatically terminate on the date of the next board meeting, when the applicant may be considered for a full and unrestricted medical license.
- Special licenses for physicians in GME programs and licenses with restrictions on practice parameters.
- Retired physician license: $50 one-time fee

Oregon
- Limited License for Institutional Practice (IP), Public Health, Visiting Professor (VP), Medical Faculty (MF), SPEX, Special, Postgraduate, and Fellow, which may be valid up to 1 year. LL-VP and Fellow licenses may be renewed for 1 additional year, LL-MF for 3 additional years.
- LL-IP good only in state institutions.
- LL-VP valid for a 1-year teaching position.
- LL-MF valid for a full-time faculty position offered by dean of medical school.
- LL-SPEX valid while awaiting results of SPEX examination.
- LL-Special allows applicant with complete file to practice between two board meetings.

Pennsylvania
- Interim Limited License (up to 12 consecutive months) to physicians providing medical service other than at the training location of the licensee's accredited GME program.
- Graduate License allows licensee to participate for a period of up to 12 consecutive months in GME within the complex of the hospital to which the licensee is assigned and any satellite facility or other training location used in the program.
- Institutional License allows qualified person to teach and/or practice medicine for a period of time not to exceed 3 years in one of the Commonwealth's medical colleges, its affiliates, or community hospitals.
- Temporary License allows licensee to teach medicine and surgery or participate in a medical procedure necessary for the well-being of a specified patient within the Common-wealth or to practice medicine and surgery at a camp or resort for no more than 3 months. Applicants for a temporary license must hold an unrestricted license in another state, territory, possession, or country.
- Extraterritorial License granted to licensed physicians maintaining an office to practice near the boundary line of an adjoining state whose medical practice extends into Pennsylvania.
- Volunteer license available for retired physicians

Table 15 (continued)
**Temporary or Limited Licenses, Permits, Certificates,
and Registration Issued by State Medical Boards**

Puerto Rico
- Internship or residency licenses to qualified applicants enrolled in an ACGME-accredited residency program who have successfully completed the first part of the medical board examination (basic sciences) or its equivalent (NBME, FLEX, or USMLE).
- Public service licenses to qualified applicants who have completed at least 1 year of accredited residency education and who have passed all three parts of the medical board examination or its equivalent (NBME, FLEX, or USMLE).

Rhode Island
- One-year limited medical registration to trainees appointed as an intern, resident, fellow, or medical officer in a hospital. Practice limited to the designated institution and must be under the supervision of a staff physician licensed in this state.
- Limited faculty license, on petition by dean.

South Carolina
- Limited licenses for residency programs or limited practices on a yearly basis.
- Temporary license to any applicant who meets all requirements pending final board approval.

South Dakota
Sixty-day locum tenens permit and resident physician license.

Texas
Physician-in-training permits to residents, interns, and fellows (these permits have requirements that gradually increase in difficulty with each renewal); temporary licenses pending final board approval.

Vermont
- Limited license to interns, residents, fellows, or house officers enrolled in an ACGME-accredited residency program and working under supervision of licensed physician at a state-licensed institution or clinic.
- Physicians appointed full-time to the faculty of the College of Medicine of the University of Vermont receive Vermont license, issued for the duration of the appointment.

Virginia
- Temporary license/certificate for continuing education, summer camps, and free clinics.
- Limited license for fellowship and teaching positions.
- Temporary licenses (renewable annually) to interns, residents, and fellows in accredited programs in Virginia.
- Retired physician license: $130 inactive reregistration fee.

Virgin Islands
- Temporary licenses (2 years) in connection with government employment only.
- Limited-scope inactive licenses (valid 30 days, nonrenewable).

Washington
- Limited license to physicians in GME and teaching/research at state institutions and city/county health departments.
- Teaching (visiting professor) license for teaching/ research at state institutions or city/county health fellowships, only to physicians currently licensed in another state or country.
- Temporary permit (valid 90 days) only in conjunction with full application; applicant must have been previously licensed in an approved state.

West Virginia
- Temporary license (valid until subsequent board meeting) after completed application for permanent license has been filed, processed, and found in order.
- IMGs must be ECFMG-certified.

Wisconsin
- Temporary educational certificates for residency education after first year; may be renewed annually for not more than 4 years.
- Camp physician's license to physicians for locum tenens or working in a camp up to 90 days.

Wyoming
Temporary license between board meetings after completed application for permanent license has been filed, processed, and approved by the board.

Note: *All information should be verified with the licensing board; medical licenses are granted to those physicians meeting all state requirements—at the discretion of the board.*

Regulations on the Practice of Telemedicine and Out-of-state Consulting Physicians

For purposes of this publication, telemedicine is defined as the delivery of health care services via electronic means from a health care provider in one location to a patient in another. Applications that fall under this definition include the transfer of medical images, such as pathology slides or radiographs, interactive video consultations between patient and provider or between primary care and specialty care physicians, and mental health consultations. Twenty-seven states have adopted regulations concerning the practice of telemedicine; 10 other states have begun to develop regulations.

Table 16
Regulations on the Practice of Telemedicine and Out-of-state Consulting Physicians

	Practice of Telemedicine		
	Has Adopted Regulations	Has Begun to Develop Regulations	Specific Licensure Restrictions on and/or Requirements for Out-of-state Consulting Physicians
Alabama	Yes		Issues a "special purpose" license (1997)
Alaska			Active Alaska license required. Exceptions are made for an MD or DO who is not a resident of Alaska and who is asked by an Alaskan MD or DO to help in the diagnosis or treatment of a case.
Arizona			No license required for single or infrequent consultation from out-of-state physician with licensed physician. Full license required of any physician providing services via technology
Arkansas	Yes		
California	Yes		No license required for consultations with a primary care physician licensed in California.
Colorado	Yes		Licensed Colorado physician may consult with physicians licensed in another state. Full license required to use telemedicine to diagnose and treat diseases.
Connecticut	Yes		No license required for any physician residing out of state who is employed to come to Connecticut to render temporary assistance to or consult with a licensed Connecticut physician.
Delaware		Yes	
DC		Yes	
Florida	Yes		Physician licensed in another state, territory, or foreign country is permitted to examine the patient, take a history and physical, review laboratory tests and x-rays, and make recommendations about diagnosis and treatment to a licensed Florida physician. The term "consultation" does not include such physician's performance of any medical procedure on or the rendering of treatment to the patient. Full licensure required for out-of-state physicians using telemedicine to treat Florida residents.
Georgia	Yes		License required for out-of-state telemedicine.
Guam			Must hold license in state where physician resides.
Hawaii	Yes		Out-of-state consultant must be licensed in the state in which he/she resides; may not open an office (or appoint a place to meet patients or receive calls) in Hawaii.
Idaho			No license required for out-of-state physicians consulted by licensed Idaho physicians. Idaho medical license *is* required if out-of-state physician is directly consulted by an Idaho patient.
Illinois	Yes		Full license required.
Indiana	Yes		
Iowa		Yes	No license required for incidental consultation with out-of-state physicians by licensed Iowa physicians; out-of-state physician must be licensed if providing medical services to Iowa patients.
Kansas	Yes		License required if orders for services are issued for individuals located in Kansas. No license required for consultant licensed in another state who does not open an office or maintain a place to meet patients or receive calls in Kansas. No license required for services performed under supervision or by order of or referral from a licensed Kansas physician.
Kentucky			No license required for single or infrequent consultation from out-of-state physician with licensed physician. Full license required of any physician providing services via technology
Louisiana			
Maine	Yes		No license required for incidental consultation with out-of-state physicians by licensed Maine physicians; out-of-state physician must be licensed if providing medical services to Maine patients.
Maryland			Maryland license required, unless in consultation with a licensed Maryland physician.
Massachusetts			
Michigan		Yes	No license required for a physician living in and authorized to practice in another state or country who, in exceptional circumstances, is called for consultation or treatment by a Michigan health professional.
Minnesota			Cannot assume primary patient care responsibility; physician of record must have Minnesota license; orders are countersigned by licensed Minnesota physician.
Mississippi	Yes		No license required for out-of-state physicians called for consultation by a licensed physician residing in Mississippi. Consultation period cannot exceed 5 days. Full license required for physicians rendering a medical opinion concerning diagnosis or treatment via electronic or other means.
Missouri	Yes		Licensed Missouri physician may consult with physicians licensed in another state. Full license required to use telemedicine to diagnose and treat diseases.

Table 16 (continued)
Regulations on the Practice of Telemedicine and Out-of-state Consulting Physicians

| | Practice of Telemedicine | | |
	Has Adopted Regulations	Has Begun to Develop Regulations	Specific Licensure Restrictions on and/or Requirements for Out-of-state Consulting Physicians
Montana	Yes		License required if an out-of-state consultant establishes a regular, direct physician/patient relationship.
Nebraska	Yes		Nonresident physicians not holding a Nebraska license cannot practice medicine, except when called in consultation by a licensed Nebraska physician.
Nevada	Yes		License required if consultant's work constitutes the practice of medicine.
New Hampshire			License required if consultation is not made directly with a licensed New Hampshire physician.
New Jersey		Yes	
New Mexico	Yes		License required for all out-of-state consultants.
New York		Yes	License in home jurisdiction required.
North Carolina	Yes		North Carolina license required.
North Dakota	Yes		
Ohio			No license required for out-of-state consultant who is licensed in another jurisdiction when in consultation with a licensed Ohio practitioner.
Oklahoma	Yes		
Oregon		Yes	Permanent license required to practice medicine.
Pennsylvania		Yes	Pennsylvania license required.
Puerto Rico			
Rhode Island		Yes	Requirements exist for out-of-state consultants.
South Carolina			Must consult with a licensed South Carolina physician.
South Dakota	Yes		Any nonresident MD or DO who, while located outside South Dakota, provides diagnostic or treatment services through electronic means to a patient in this state under a contract with a health care provider, a clinic in this state that provides health services, or health care facility is engaged in the practice of medicine or osteopathy in South Dakota. Out-of-state MDs or DOs who consult on an irregular basis with a licensed South Dakota physician are not considered to practice in South Dakota.
Tennessee	Yes		Telemedicine license required of out-of-state physicians diagnosing or treating patients in Tennessee. Some exceptions granted.
Texas	Yes		Special Purpose License required for practice of medicine across state lines.
Utah	Yes		No license required of out-of-state physicians consulting with licensed Utah physician; full license required if consulting directly with patient by any means.
Vermont			
Virgin Islands			
Virginia			Virginia license required if practice of medicine occurs in state.
Washington			May not set up an office, appoint a place of meeting patients, or receive calls within this state.
West Virginia	Yes		License required (with exceptions).
Wisconsin		Yes	
Wyoming	Yes		No license required of physicians residing in and licensed to practice medicine in another state or country called for consultation via telephone, electronic, or any other means by a licensed Wyoming physician. License required if consultations exceed one 7-day period in any 52-week period.
Total	**27**	**10**	

Note: *All information should be verified with the licensing board; medical licenses are granted to those physicians meeting all state requirements—at the discretion of the board.*

Section II.

Medical Licensing Examinations and Organizations

The United States Medical Licensing Examination™ (USMLE)™ *

*Office of the USMLE Secretariat,
Philadelphia, Pennsylvania*

The United States Medical Licensing Examination (USMLE) is a three-step examination for medical licensure in the United States sponsored by the following organizations:

- Federation of State Medical Boards (FSMB)
- National Board of Medical Examiners® (NBME®)

The Composite Committee, appointed by the FSMB and NBME, governs the USMLE. The Composite Committee establishes rules for the USMLE program. Membership includes representatives from the following:

- FSMB
- NBME
- Educational Commission for Foreign Medical Graduates (ECFMG®)
- American public

In the United States and its territories, the individual medical licensing authorities ("state medical boards") of the various jurisdictions grant a license to practice medicine. Each medical licensing authority sets its own rules and regulations and requires passing an examination that demonstrates qualification for licensure. Results of the USMLE are reported to these authorities for use in granting the initial license to practice medicine. The USMLE provides them with a common evaluation system for applicants for medical licensure. Because individual medical licensing authorities make their own decisions regarding use of USMLE results, licensure applicants should obtain complete information from the licensing authority. The FSMB can also provide general information on medical licensure.

Step 1, Step 2, and Step 3 of the USMLE

The USMLE is designed to assess a physician's ability to apply knowledge, concepts, and principles that are important in health and disease and that constitute the basis of safe and effective patient care. The USMLE is a single examination with three Steps. Each Step is complementary to the others; no Step can stand alone in the assessment of readiness for medical licensure.

Step 1 assesses whether medical school students or graduates can understand and apply important concepts of the sciences basic to the practice of medicine, with special emphasis on principles and mechanisms underlying health, disease, and modes of therapy. Step 1 ensures mastery of not only the sciences underlying the safe and competent practice of medicine in the present, but also the scientific principles required for maintenance of competence through lifelong learning.

Step 2 assesses whether medical school students or graduates can apply the medical knowledge and understanding of clinical science considered essential for the provision of patient care under supervision, including emphasis on health promotion and disease prevention. The inclusion of Step 2 in the USMLE sequence is intended to ensure that due attention is devoted to principles of clinical science that undergird the safe and competent practice of medicine.

Step 3 assesses whether physicians can apply the medical knowledge and understanding of biomedical and clinical science considered essential for the unsupervised practice of medicine, with emphasis on patient management in ambulatory settings. The inclusion of Step 3 in the USMLE sequence ensures that attention is devoted to the importance of assessing the knowledge of physicians who are assuming independent responsibility for delivering general medical care to patients.

* Portions reprinted with permission from the *USMLE 2001 Bulletin of Information*, copyright © 2000 by the Federation of State Medical Boards of the United States, Inc, and the National Board of Medical Examiners; and also from *1999 Annual Report*, copyright © 2000 by the National Board of Medical Examiners.

USMLE Eligibility Requirements and Examination Policies

To be eligible to sit for USMLE Step 1 or Step 2, an applicant must be in one of the following categories at the time of application and on the examination day:

- a medical student officially enrolled in, or a graduate of, a United States or Canadian medical school program leading to the MD degree that is accredited by the Liaison Committee on Medical Education (LCME)

- a medical student officially enrolled in, or a graduate of, a United States medical school that is accredited by the American Osteopathic Association (AOA)

- a medical student officially enrolled in, or a graduate of, a foreign medical school and eligible for examination by the ECFMG for its certificate

To be eligible to sit for USMLE Step 3, an applicant must meet all of the following require-ments:

- Meet the requirements for taking Step 3 imposed by the medical licensing authority sponsoring the exam.

- Obtain the MD degree (or its equivalent) or the DO degree.

- Obtain passing scores on both Steps 1 and 2.

- If a graduate of a foreign medical school, obtain certification by the ECFMG or successfully complete a Fifth Pathway program (see p. 23 for more information).

The USMLE program recommends that for Step 3 eligibility licensing authorities require the completion, or near completion, of at least 1 postgraduate training year in a graduate medical education program accredited by the Accreditation Council for Graduate Medical Education (ACGME) or the AOA. Applicants should contact the FSMB or the individual licensing authority for complete information on Step 3 eligibility requirements in the state where they plan to be licensed.

Medical students or graduates planning to take the USMLE must obtain the most recent information from the appropriate registration entity before applying for the examination. See the USMLE Web site (www.usmle.org) for updated information.

Computer-based Testing (CBT)

The USMLE is administered by computer. Prometric, Inc®, a subsidiary of Thomson Learning™, provides scheduling and test centers for the USMLE. Step 1 and Step 2 examinations are given around the world at Prometric test centers. Step 3 is given at Prometric test centers in the United States and its territories. To take a USMLE Step, medical students or graduates must meet the eligibility requirements and do the following:

- Obtain application materials from, and then complete and submit the materials to, the appropriate registration entity.

- Receive a Scheduling Permit verifying eligibility and authorizing the applicant to schedule the examination.

- Follow the instructions on the Scheduling Permit to schedule test date(s) at a specific Prometric test center.

- On the scheduled date(s) and at the scheduled time, bring to the Prometric test center the Scheduling Permit and the required identification described on it, and take the test.

Description of the Examinations

The examinations are administered in sessions of 8 or 9 hours, broken up into sections, or "blocks." The computer keeps track of overall session time, including break time and time allocated for each block of the test.

Step 1

Step 1 has approximately 350 multiple-choice test items, divided into seven 60-minute blocks, administered in one 8-hour testing session.

Step 1 includes test questions in anatomy, behavioral sciences, biochemistry, microbiology, pathology, pharmacology, and physiology, as well as interdisciplinary topics such as nutrition, genetics, and aging. Step 1 is a broadly based, integrated examination. Test questions commonly require examinees to interpret graphic and tabular material, to identify gross and microscopic pathologic and normal specimens, and to apply basic science knowledge to clinical problems. Step 1 is constructed according to an integrated content outline that organizes basic science material along two dimensions: system and process. Further information on examination content and sample Step 1 test materials are made available when applicants register for the examination and at the USMLE Web site (www.usmle.org).

Step 2

Step 2 has approximately 400 multiple-choice test items, divided into eight 60-minute blocks, administered in one 9-hour testing session.

Step 2 includes test questions in internal medicine, obstetrics and gynecology, pediatrics, preventive medicine, psychiatry, surgery, and other areas relevant to provision of care under supervision. The majority of the test questions describe clinical situations and require providing a diagnosis, a prognosis, an indication of underlying mechanisms of disease, or the next step in medical care, including preventive measures. Step 2 is a broadly based, integrated examination. Interpretation of tables and laboratory data, imaging studies, photographs of gross and microscopic pathologic specimens, and results of other diagnostic studies is frequently required.

Step 2 is constructed according to an integrated content outline that organizes clinical science material along two dimensions: physician task and disease process. Further information on examination content and sample Step 2 test materials are made available when applicants register for the examination and at the USMLE Web site (www.usmle.org).

Step 3

Step 3 has approximately 500 multiple-choice test items, divided into blocks of 25 to 50 items, and approximately nine computer-based case simulations, taken in blocks of one or more cases. Between 30 and 60 minutes is provided to complete each block. Step 3 is administered in two 8-hour testing sessions.

Step 3 is organized along two principal dimensions: clinical encounter frame and physician task. Step 3 content reflects a data-based model of generalist medical practice in the United States.

Encounter frames capture the essential features of circumstances surrounding physicians' clinical activity with patients. They range from encounters with patients seen for the first time for nonemergency problems, to encounters with regular patients seen in the context of continued care, to patient encounters in (life-threatening) emergency situations. Encounters occur in clinics, offices, nursing homes, hospitals, emergency departments, and on the telephone. Each test item in an encounter frame also represents one of the six physician tasks. For example, initial care encounters emphasize taking a history and performing a physical examination. In contrast, continued care encounters emphasize decisions regarding prognosis and management.

High-frequency, high-impact diseases also organize the content of Step 3. Clinician experts assign clinical problems related to these diseases to individual clinical encounter frames to represent their occurrence in generalist practice.

Step 3 includes Primum® computer-based case simulations (CCS), a test format developed by the NBME that allows the medical student or physician taking the test to provide care for a simulated patient. The test-taker decides which diagnostic information to obtain and how to treat and monitor the patient's progress. The computer records each step taken in caring for the patient and scores overall performance. This format permits assessment of clinical decision-making skills in a more realistic and integrated manner than other available formats.

In Primum CCS, the test-taker may request information from the history and physical examination; order laboratory studies, procedures, and consultants; and start medications and other therapies. Any of the thousands of possible entries that are typed on the "order sheet" are processed and verified by the "clerk." When the test-taker has confirmed that there is nothing further to do, he or she decides when to reevaluate the patient by advancing time. As time passes, the patient's condition changes based on the underlying problem and interventions taken; results of tests are reported and results of interventions must be monitored. The test-taker can suspend the movement of time to consider next steps. While one cannot go back in time, orders can be changed to reflect an updated management plan.

The patient's chart contains, in addition to the order sheet, the reports resulting from orders. By selecting the appropriate chart tabs, the test-taker can review vital signs, progress notes, nurses' notes, and test results. He or she may care for and move the patient among the office, home, emergency department, intensive care unit, and hospital ward.

Preparation for the Examinations

No test preparation courses are affiliated with or sanctioned by the USMLE program. Information on such courses is not available from the ECFMG, FSMB, NBME, USMLE Secretariat, or medical licensing authorities.

USMLE Steps are broad in scope and are designed to measure the prospective physician's ability to apply knowledge. The best preparation for the USMLE is a general, thorough review of the content reflected in the materials for each Step which are provided to applicants when they register.

Sample test materials to practice with the testing software are provided to eligible applicants from their registration entity and are available at the USMLE Web site. The NBME provides students and graduates of accredited medical schools in the United States with a compact disc (CD) that includes sample test materials. Applicants should run the sample test materials and acquaint themselves with the software well before their test date(s). Practice time is not available on the test day. A brief tutorial on the test day provides a review of the test software, including navigation tools and examination format, prior to beginning the test. It does not provide an opportunity to practice.

Physicians taking Step 3 must practice with the Primum software well in advance of the test. Experience has shown that those who do not practice with the format and mechanics of managing the patients in Primum CCS are likely to be at a disadvantage when taking the cases under standardized test conditions. Extensive practice time is not available on the test day. Step 3 applicants must review the Primum CCS orientation materials and practice with all the practice cases prior to their testing day to have a thorough understanding of how the CCS system works. The CCS software is included on the USMLE CD provided in Step 3 application materials. The CD is also sent to LCME- and AOA-accredited medical schools and residency training programs. The CCS practice cases can also be obtained from the USMLE Web site.

Examination Performance

The implementation of computer-based testing changed the nature and timing of the examinee cohorts. As a result, performance information listed here includes only the final paper-and-pencil tests. No Step 1 scores are reported because no paper-and-pencil tests were administered during 1999, and data for the initial full-year cohort of Step 1 examinees who completed testing in April 2000 are not yet available. Step 2 performance information for the August 1998 and March 1999 administrations and Step 3 performance information for the May 1999 administration are shown in Tables 17-18.

While the first CBT examinee cohorts for Step 1 and Step 2 are not included, performance for US Step 1 and Step 2 examinees was similar to prior years, based on the 25,926 Step 1 examinees and 10,415 Step 2 examinees for whom scores were reported by December 31, 1999. Only about half as many students and graduates of foreign medical schools took Step 1 and Step 2 during 1999 as in 1997. The students and graduates of foreign medical schools who were tested performed somewhat better on average than the larger group in past years. The decline in numbers of examinees from foreign medical schools began in 1998.

While the Step 3 cohort will not be complete until the end of 2000, initial results based upon the scores of approximately 7500 Step 3 examinees reported in April 2000 appear to be comparable to prior years.

Reporting of cohort performance information for all three Steps will resume when it becomes available.

Table 17
1998-1999 USMLE Step 2 Administrations: Number Tested and Percent Passing

	August 1998		March 1999		Total 1998-1999	
	# Tested	% Passing	# Tested	% Passing	# Tested	% Passing
US/Canadian Examinees						
Allopathic Students	11,745	93%	6,248	91%	17,993	92%
First-time Takers	11,079	95%	5,450	94%	16,529	95%
Repeaters	666	55%	798	67%	1,464	62%
Osteopathic Students	64	78%	79	86%	143	83%
First-time Takers	56	82%	73	88%	129	85%
Repeaters	8	50%	6	67%	14	57%
Total US/Canadian	*11,809*	*93%*	*6,327*	*91%*	*18,136*	*92%*
IMG Registrants*						
First-time Takers	4,068	56%	4,060	62%	8,128	59%
Repeaters	4,328	32%	4,436	42%	8,764	37%
Total IMG	*8,396*	*44%*	*8,496*	*52%*	*16,892*	*48%*

* For IMG examinees, first-time takers are defined as examinees who had not taken Part II or Step 2 previously; repeaters are defined as examinees who had taken Part II or Step 2 previously. The first-time taker group includes a small percentage of examinees who had taken the Foreign Medical Graduate Examination in the Medical Sciences (FMGEMS) prior to its discontinuation in 1993 but had not yet taken Part II or Step 2.

Table 18
1999 USMLE Step 3 Administrations: Number Tested and Percent Passing

	May 1999	
	# Tested	% Passing
Graduates of US or Canadian Schools		
Allopathic Students	10,662	92%
First-time Takers	9,995	95%
Repeaters*	667	56%
Osteopathic Students	45	87%
First-time Takers	44	86%
Repeaters*	1	**
Total US/Canadian Graduates	*10,707*	*92%*
Graduates of Foreign Medical Schools		
First-time Takers	3,794	56%
Repeaters	3,198	38%
Total International Medical Graduates	*6,992*	*48%*

*Repeaters are those with any prior attempt at Step 3, NBME Part III, or FLEX Component 2.

**Performance data not reported for categories containing fewer than five examinees.

Communicating About USMLE

Examination	Type of Applicant	Entity to Contact
Step 1 or Step 2	Students and graduates of accredited medical schools in the United States and Canada	NBME Department of Licensing Examination Services 3750 Market St Philadelphia, PA 19104-3190 215 590-9700 215 590-9457 Fax www.nbme.org
Step 1 or Step 2	Students and graduates of medical schools outside the US, Canada, and Puerto Rico	ECFMG 3624 Market St Philadelphia, PA 19104-2685 Application materials: www.ecfmg.org 215 375-1913 800 500-8249 toll-free Other inquiries: 215 386-5900 215 387-9963 Fax
Step 3	All medical school graduates who have passed Step 1 and Step 2	Medical licensing authority – or – FSMB Dept of Examination Services 400 Fuller Wiser Rd/Ste 300 Euless, TX 76039-3855 817 868-4041 www.fsmb.org

Complete information on the USMLE is available at the USMLE Web site. General inquiries regarding the USMLE may be directed to:

USMLE Secretariat
3750 Market St
Philadelphia, PA 19104-3190
215 590-9600

The Federation of State Medical Boards of the United States, Inc.

Founded in 1912, the Federation of State Medical Boards of the United States, Inc (FSMB) is a nonprofit organization composed of the 69 allopathic, osteopathic, and composite medical licensing boards of all the states, the District of Columbia, Guam, Puerto Rico, and the Virgin Islands.

The primary responsibility of each medical licensing board is to protect the public through the regulation of physicians and other health care providers. Within the United States, the organization and activities of each board are determined by state statute, usually referred to as a medical practice act. In general, each state medical board has the authority to license physicians, regulate the practice of medicine, and discipline those who violate the medical practice act.

The FSMB serves as a liaison, advocate, researcher, and educator and information source to the public, to health care organizations, and to state, national, and international authorities. It works to improve the quality, safety, and integrity of US health care by promoting high standards for physician licensure and practice and assisting and supporting state medical boards in regulating medical practice and protecting the public.

FSMB Services

The FSMB provides the following services designed to assist member medical boards in their role as public protectors.

Board Action Data Bank

A central repository for formal actions taken against physicians by state licensing and disciplinary boards, Canadian licensing authorities, the US armed forces, the US Department of Health and Human Services, and other regulatory bodies, the Data Bank contains more than 75,000 prejudicial and nonprejudicial actions related to approximately 30,000 physicians. This information is available to licensing and disciplinary boards; military,

governmental, and private agencies; and physician credentialing organizations.

Licensure and Assessment Services

In the United States and its territories, a license to practice medicine is a privilege granted only by the individual medical licensing authority of a state or jurisdiction. Each authority sets its own rules and regulations, and each requires successful completion of an examination or certification demonstrating qualification for licensure.

The FSMB, in collaboration with the National Board of Medical Examiners (see p. 63), offers two service packages used by medical licensing authorities for making licensure decisions: The United States Medical Licensing Examination (USMLE™) and the Post-Licensure Assessment System (PLAS).

USMLE

The USMLE is a 3-step examination taken by individuals preparing for initial medical licensure in the United States. With steps designed to be taken at different times during medical education and training, the USMLE provides a single pathway for evaluating an individual's ability to apply medical knowledge, concepts and principles to patient care (see p. 54 for more information on USMLE).

Post-Licensure Assessment System (PLAS)

The Post-Licensure Assessment System (PLAS) is a joint program of the FSMB and the National Board of Medical Examiners (NBME). The PLAS is intended to provide comprehensive services to medical licensing authorities for use in assessing the ongoing competency of licensed physicians. PLAS comprises two independent yet complementary programs: the Special Purpose Examination (SPEX) program and the Assessment Center Program. Collectively, they provide a standardized, national program for assisting state medical boards in ensuring that qualified, competent physicians are licensed to practice medicine.

Federation Credentials Verification Service (FCVS)

The Federation Credentials Verification Service (FCVS) was launched in September 1996 to provide a centralized, uniform process for state medical boards to obtain a verified, primary-source record of a physician's medical credentials. This service is designed to lighten the workload of credentialing staff and reduce duplication of effort by gathering, verifying, and permanently storing the physician's credentials in a central repository at the Federation's offices. FCVS obtains primary source verification of medical education, postgraduate training, examination history, board action history, and identity. This repository of information allows a physician to establish a confidential, lifetime professional portfolio with FCVS which can be forwarded, at the physician's request, to any state medical board that has established an agreement with FCVS—as well as private, governmental, and commercial entities.

To request an FCVS application, receive more detailed information about the credentialing process, or request a roster of the state medical boards that accept FCVS documents, call toll-free 888 ASK-FCVS (888 275-3287), access the federation Web site at www.fsmb.org, or send an e-mail to fcvs@fsmb.org.

Legislative Services

The Federation monitors federal and state legislation and regulatory policies that affect medical regulation. Legislative Services attempts to identify current legislative trends and facilitates communication among member medical boards on issues of mutual interest. Legislative Services assists member boards in legislative and administrative efforts to implement Federation policy initiatives through formal policy statements, research assistance, written or oral testimony, letters to legislative leadership, etc. The Federation has played a key role in state and national debates on many prominent issues, including telemedicine, Internet prescribing, physician profiling, management of chronic pain, oversight of resident physicians, managed care, and reduction of medical errors.

Publications

The FSMB publishes several monthly and quarterly publications, committee reports, and other medical regulation and licensure-related publications/documents. These publications provide information on current trends in medical regulation and licensure, position statements, and policies on issues that affect the FSMB and its member boards.

Education

The FSMB education department offers various educational programs to its members, including the Annual Meeting, Board Investigator Workshops, Regional Workshops, Board Attorney's Workshop, Executive Management Seminar, New Executives Orientation, and Senior Executive Certification Program. CME and CLE are also available through various program offerings.

Library Services

The Library Services department provides research assistance to member boards and the general public on topical issues dealing with medical licensure and discipline. Nonmember library research requests are based on an hourly charge of $35.

Post-Licensure Assessment System (PLAS)

Established in 1998 by the FSMB and the NBME, the Post-Licensure Assessment System (PLAS) offers two services to assist state medical boards in assessing a licensed physicians competency to practice medicine: the Special Purpose Examination (SPEX) and the Assessment Center Program. The purpose of SPEX is to provide a high-quality, objective, and standardized cognitive examination as a tool to assess current knowledge requisite for general, undifferentiated medical practice by physicians who hold or who have held a valid, unrestricted license in a US or Canadian jurisdiction. The Assessment Center Program is intended to provide a personalized, multimodal evaluation of a licensed physician's competence to practice medicine as well as recommendations for remediation.

Special Purpose Examination (SPEX)

SPEX is available to licensing boards for reexamination of physicians for whom the board determines the need for a demonstration of current medical knowledge. These may include physicians seeking licensure reinstatement or reactivation after some period of professional inactivity due to chronic illness, raising a family, recovering from some impairment or for a physician involved in a disciplinary proceeding in which the board determined the need for evaluation. The SPEX is also appropriate for physicians applying for licensure by endorsement who are some years beyond initial examination. Physicians who hold a current, unrestricted license to practice medicine in a US or Canadian jurisdiction are also able to apply for SPEX as a self-nominated candidate, independent of any request or approval from a medical licensing board.

A guiding design principle is that SPEX content should reflect the knowledge and cognitive abilities required of all physicians, regardless of specialty practiced. The questions used in SPEX focus on a core of clinical knowledge and relevant underlying basic science principles deemed necessary to form a reasonable foundation for the safe and effective practice of medicine. Specifically, there are two primary dimensions of the SP EX: clinical encounter categories (well-care/preventive medicine; acute, circumscribed problems; ill-defined presentations or problems; chronic or progressive illness; emergency conditions, critical care; and behavioral/emotional problems) and physician tasks (data gathering, diagnostic assessment, managing therapy, and applying scientific concepts). This principle reflects the fact that unrestricted licensure in the United States is for the "practice of medicine," not for the practice of a particular specialty.

SPEX is a 1-day, computer-administered examination consisting of 420 multiple-choice questions in two sections of 3 hours and 15 minutes each and is administered through Prometric test centers in coordination with the NBME. Prometric offers test sites across the United State, its territories, Canada, Puerto Rico, and the Virgin Islands. For a more detailed list of testing centers, refer to www.prometric.com. SPEX scores are reported on a two-digit scale by which a score of 75 is the minimum passpoint recommended for use by licensing boards. SPEX scores are initially reported directly to the licensing boards for which SPEX is taken and/or the examinee. The FSMB maintains a data bank of all SPEX scores to facilitate interstate endorsement. As it does for FLEX and USMLE, the FSMB will provide certified transcripts of SPEX scores to licensing boards receiving license applications from individuals taking SPEX in other jurisdictions.

Assessment Services

As of April 1, 2000, medical licensing boards have access to a new service to assist them in their evaluation of physicians with clinical performance issues. A program of extensive diagnostic assessments is being offered through the combined efforts of the FSMB and the NBME. Assessments are made in areas of record keeping, clinical knowledge, patient management skills, clinical and communications skills, cognitive functioning, and clinical reasoning. Test instruments include standardized, computer-based case simulations and a multiple-choice examination. Other standardized and personalized procedures are also incorporated, including chart-stimulated recall interviews and simulated patients. The testing period is 2 to 3 days.

The assessment focuses on identifying the client physician's strengths and opportunities for improvement. This information is summarized in a narrative report provided to the physician and the referring state medical board. The report contains descriptive data detailing the results of the individual's assessment and provides recommendations for remediation of the physician's deficient areas. The state medical boards can use the assessment report as a tool in their decision-making process and, if necessary, in formulating appropriate remediation recommendations for the physician.

Assessment services are provided through the Colorado Personalized Education for Physicians (CPEP) program, which has been active in assessing physicians for 10 years.

Information

Federation of State Medical Boards of the United States
400 Fuller Wiser Rd/Ste 300
Euless, TX 76039
817 868-4000
817 868-4099 Fax
www.fsmb.org

National Board of Medical Examiners

The National Board of Medical Examiners® (NBME®), together with the Federation of State Medical Boards as the parent organizations of the United States Medical Licensing Examination™ (USMLE™), develop the three-step United States Medical Licensing Examination. The USMLE provides a common evaluation system for applicants seeking initial licensure to practice medicine in the United States. The examination is designed to assess a physician's ability to apply knowledge, concepts, and principles that are important in health and disease and that constitute the basis of safe and effective patient care. For more information on the USMLE, see p. 54.

In 1999, computer-based testing was phased in for USMLE Step 1, Step 2, and Step 3 examinations. Accordingly, the final paper and pencil administrations of Step 2 and Step 3 were in March 1999 and May 1999, respectively (no paper and pencil administration of Step 1 was given in 1999). Computer-based testing began for Step 1 in May, for Step 2 in August, and for Step 3 in November. With full implementation successfully completed by the end of 1999, computer-based Step 1, Step 2, and Step 3 examinations are now offered throughout the year.

The NBME registers applicants who are students or graduates of US and Canadian medical schools accredited by the Liaison Committee on Medical Education or the American Osteopathic Association for USMLE Steps 1 and 2. Sylvan Prometric™, a division of Sylvan® Learning Systems, provided scheduling and test centers for computer-based USMLE test administrations in 1999.

Performance information for 1999 has been published only for the final Step 2 and Step 3 paper and pencil tests, as shown in Tables 17 and 18 in the USMLE Report on p. 54.

NBME Certification and Endorsements

The NBME developed and administered its own three-part examination as part of the National Board Certification Program until it was discontinued with the implementation of the USMLE.

Certification was awarded to physicians who

1. received the MD degree from an LCME-accredited medical school;

2. passed at least one NBME Part or Step examination prior to December 31, 1994; and

3. completed, with a satisfactory record, 1 full year (12 months) in a GME program accredited by the Accreditation Council for Graduate Medical Education (ACGME). Accredited internships in Canada were also recognized as meeting this requirement.

Certification by the NBME continues to be used for licensure in the United States for those physicians certified as diplomates prior to implementation of the USMLE and for examinees certified as diplomates who took a combination of NBME and/or USMLE examinations and passed at least one Part or Step prior to December 31, 1994. The last regular administration of Part I occurred in 1991, Part II in April 1992, and Part III in May 1994.

Because some medical students and physicians completed some part of the NBME examination sequence before the implementation of USMLE, certain combinations of examinations may be considered by medical licensing authorities as comparable to existing examinations. Examinees who passed a combination of examinations should obtain information regarding the acceptability of the combination directly from the medical licensing authority in the jurisdiction where the examinee plans to seek licensure.

NBME Certificates and Endorsements

In 1999, the NBME awarded a total of 446 Diplomate certificates, and NBME Diplomates requested 12,388 endorsements of record of certification to state medical licensing authorities.

For further information on USMLE examinations and on NBME certification, contact:

Department of Licensing Examination Services
National Board of Medical Examiners
3750 Market St
Philadelphia, PA 19104
215 590-9700
www.nbme.org

Section III.

Information for International Medical Graduates

Educational Commission for Foreign Medical Graduates

Stephen S. Seeling, JD
Vice President for Operations
Educational Commission for Foreign Medical Graduates
Philadelphia, Pennsylvania

The Educational Commission for Foreign Medical Graduates (ECFMG®*), through its program of certification, assesses the readiness of graduates of foreign medical schools to enter residency or fellowship programs in the United States that are accredited by the Accreditation Council for Graduate Medical Education (ACGME).

The ECFMG and its sponsoring organizations define a graduate of a foreign medical school as a physician who received his/her basic medical degree or qualification from a medical school located outside the United States, Canada, and Puerto Rico. The medical school must be listed in the World Directory of Medical Schools, published by the World Health Organization, at the time of the physician's graduation. US citizens who have completed their medical education in schools outside the United States, Canada, and Puerto Rico are considered graduates of foreign medical schools; non-US citizens who have graduated from medical schools in the United States, Canada, and Puerto Rico are not considered graduates of foreign medical schools.

ECFMG certification assures directors of ACGME-accredited residency and fellowship programs, and the people of the United States, that graduates of foreign medical schools have met minimum standards of eligibility required to enter such programs. ECFMG certification does not, however, guarantee that such graduates will be accepted into these programs, since the number of applicants often exceeds the number of available positions.

ECFMG certification is one of the eligibility requirements to take Step 3 of the United States Medical Licensing Examination (USMLE). Most states in the United States also require ECFMG certification to obtain licensure to practice medicine.

* The terms "ECFMG" and "CSA" are registered in the US Patent and Trademark Office.

ECFMG Certification Requirements

To be eligible for ECFMG certification, international medical graduates must meet the following requirements:

Examination Requirements

1. Pass the basic medical and clinical science components of the medical science examination within a 7-year period. USMLE Step 1 (basic medical) and Step 2 (clinical) are currently administered to meet this requirement.**

ECFMG accepts a passing performance on former medical science examinations for the purpose of ECFMG certification. Those formerly administered by ECFMG are:

- ECFMG Examination

- Visa Qualifying Examination (VQE)

- Foreign Medical Graduate Examination in the Medical Sciences (FMGEMS)

- Part I and Part II Examinations of the National Board of Medical Examiners (NBME)

Combinations of exams are also acceptable. Specifically, applicants who have passed only part of the former VQE, FMGEMS, or the NBME Part I or Part II may combine a passing performance on the basic medical science component of one of these exams or USMLE Step 1 with a passing performance on the clinical science component of one of the other exams or USMLE Step 2, provided that

** This policy applies only to ECFMG certification. The USMLE program has made specific recommendations to medical licensing authorities regarding the time to complete all three Steps and the number of attempts allowed to pass each Step. Applicants who are taking the Steps for the purpose of licensure should refer to *Time Limit and Number of Attempts Allowed to Complete All Steps, Formerly Administered Examinations and Retakes* in the USMLE *Bulletin of Information* for more information. Applicants should also contact the medical licensing authority of the jurisdiction where they plan to apply for licensure or the FSMB, since licensure requirements vary among jurisdictions.

the components are passed within the period specified for the exam program. Additionally, ECFMG accepts, for the purpose of its certification, a score of 75 or higher on each of the 3 days of a single administration of the former Federation Licensing Examination (FLEX), if taken prior to June 1985.**

2. Pass the English language proficiency test. There are two ways to satisfy the English language proficiency requirement for ECFMG certification. A passing performance on the former ECFMG English Test, which was administered for the last time on March 3, 1999, is accepted by ECFMG to meet this requirement. Applicants who have not passed the former ECFMG English Test can satisfy the English language proficiency requirement by achieving a score acceptable to ECFMG on the Test of English as a Foreign Language (TOEFL). These applicants may take either a computer-based administration or a paper-based, Friday or Saturday (formerly special or international) administration of TOEFL. Applicants who have never taken the ECFMG English Test must pass the TOEFL on or after March 4, 1999, to satisfy this requirement. Passing performance on either test is valid for 2 years from the date passed for the purpose of entry into graduate medical education.

3. Pass the Clinical Skills Assessment (CSA$^{®*}$). The CSA is a 1-day exam that requires examinees to demonstrate both clinical proficiency and spoken English language proficiency. The CSA is administered throughout the year at the ECFMG Clinical Skills Assessment Center in Philadelphia, Pennsylvania. Passing performance on the CSA is valid for 3 years from the date passed for the purpose of entry into graduate medical education.

Medical Education Credential Requirements

4. Document the completion of all requirements for, and receipt of, the final medical diploma. All graduates of foreign medical schools must have had at least 4 credit years (academic years for which credit has been given toward completion of the medical curriculum) in attendance at a medical school listed in the *World Directory of*

Medical Schools at the time of graduation. (The *Directory* is published by the World Health Organization, which is not an accrediting agency. It contains information supplied by countries about their medical schools. If a country or medical school that was listed in the *Directory* is removed from the *Directory*, the ECFMG Board of Trustees will give consideration on a case-by-case basis.) All documents provided to ECFMG are sent for verification to appropriate officials of the foreign medical schools.

Standard ECFMG Certificate

The ECFMG issues the Standard ECFMG Certificate to applicants who meet all of the examination and medical education credential requirements. Applicants must also pay any outstanding charges on their ECFMG financial accounts before their certificates are issued. Standard ECFMG Certificates are sent approximately 2 weeks after all of these requirements have been met.

A Standard ECFMG Certificate includes

- the name of the applicant;
- the applicant's USMLE/ECFMG Identification Number;
- the dates that examination requirements were met;
- the date that the certificate was issued;
- the date through which the passing performance on the English test remains valid for the purpose of entry into graduate medical education; and,
- the date through which the passing performance on the CSA, if required for ECFMG certification, remains valid for the purpose of entry into graduate medical education.

Certificate Revalidation Policy

Two of the exam dates on the Standard ECFMG Certificate are subject to expiration for the purpose of entering graduate medical education programs. The English test date is valid for 2 years from the most recent date of passing performance. The Clinical Skills Assessment date is valid for 3 years from the most recent date of passing performance. If the English test date has expired, an applicant will be required to demonstrate a

** This policy applies only to ECFMG certification. As of December 31, 1999, use of the former Federation Licensing Examination components or the former NBME certifying exams to fulfill eligibility requirements for Step 3 is no longer accepted. Applicants taking the Steps for the purpose of licensure should refer to *Formerly Administered Examinations* in the USMLE *Bulletin of Information*. Applicants should also contact the medical licensing authority of the jurisdiction where they plan to apply for licensure or the FSMB for specific information on licensure requirements.

performance acceptable to the ECFMG on TOEFL before entering a graduate medical education program. If the CSA date has expired, an applicant will be required to pass a subsequent CSA before entering a graduate medical education program. Once these exam requirements are met, a revalidation sticker for the appropriate examination is sent to the applicant to be affixed to the Standard ECFMG Certificate. Each revalidation sticker is unique to the individual applicant and includes the same identification number that is on the Standard ECFMG Certificate.

If an applicant's English test/CSA date(s) expire before the applicant's Standard ECFMG Certificate is issued, the applicant may revalidate these dates, as described above, prior to becoming certified by ECFMG. In this event, the English test/CSA valid-through date(s) on the Standard ECFMG Certificate will reflect the applicant's most recent passing performances on these exams.

After an applicant enters an ACGME-accredited program of graduate medical education in the United States, the applicant can request permanent validation of the Standard ECFMG Certificate. This means that the English test and CSA dates are no longer subject to expiration. To request permanent validation, the applicant and an authorized official of the training institution must complete the *Request for Permanent Validation of Standard ECFMG Certificate* (Form 246) and send it to ECFMG. After ECFMG receives and verifies the information contained on the form, a sticker indicating *valid indefinitely* status will be mailed to the applicant to be affixed to the Standard ECFMG Certificate. Each permanent validation sticker is unique to the individual applicant and includes the same identification number that is on the Standard ECFMG Certificate.

Medical Science Examination

The ECFMG requires a passing score on both a basic medical science test and a clinical science test to meet the medical science examination requirement for ECFMG certification. Step 1 (basic medical) and Step 2 (clinical) of the USMLE are currently administered to meet this requirement.

Step 1 and Step 2 of the USMLE

The USMLE is a single, three-step exam for medical licensure in the United States that provides a common system to evaluate applicants for medical licensure. The USMLE is sponsored by the Federation of State Medical Boards of the United States (FSMB) and the NBME. The USMLE is governed by a committee consisting of members of the FSMB, NBME, ECFMG, and the American public. The USMLE Steps 1, 2, and 3 replaced FLEX and the NBME Parts I, II, and III.

Step 1 assesses whether an applicant understands and can apply important science concepts basic to the practice of medicine, with special emphasis on principles and mechanisms underlying health, disease, and modes of therapy.

Step 2 assesses whether an applicant can apply the medical knowledge and understanding of clinical science essential for providing patient care under supervision, including emphasis on health promotion and disease prevention.

The ECFMG determines whether students/graduates of foreign medical schools are eligible to take USMLE Step 1 and Step 2 and registers eligible applicants to take these exams for the purpose of ECFMG certification. The NBME registers eligible students/graduates of US and Canadian medical schools accredited by the Liaison Committee on Medical Education or the American Osteopathic Association to take Step 1 and Step 2.

In 1999, the USMLE was converted from paper and pencil format to computer-based format. Computer-based Step 1 and Step 2 are delivered throughout the year by Prometric, Inc®, a subsidiary of Thomson Learning™, in its worldwide network of test centers.

English Language Proficiency Test

Physicians who assume patient care responsibilities in graduate medical education programs in the United States must be proficient in the English language. Proficiency in English is also one of the requirements for obtaining a visa to enter the United States. As a result, applicants for ECFMG certification are required to demonstrate competence in the English language.

Table 19
Examinee Performance on USMLE Step 2 Examinations and ECFMG English Tests Administered by the ECFMG in 1999

	USMLE Step 2 March 1999			ECFMG English Test March 1999		
	Number Taken	Number Passing	% Passing	Number Taken	Number Passing	% Passing
Total	8,496	4,387	51.6	6,875	4,659	67.8
First-time Takers	1,636	883	54.0	3,961	2,959	74.7
Repeaters	6,860	3,504	51.1	2,914	1,700	58.3
US Citizens	1,277	578	45.3	1,103	1,041	94.4
First-time Takers	80	31	38.8	930	901	96.9
Repeaters	1,197	547	45.7	173	140	80.9
Foreign Citizens	7,219	3,809	52.8	5,772	3,618	62.7
First-time Takers	1,556	852	54.8	3,031	2,058	67.9
Repeaters	5,663	2,957	52.2	2,741	1,560	56.9

Notes: *First-time Takers are those examinees with no prior ECFMG, VQE, FMGEMS, NBME Part I and Part II, or USMLE Step 1 and Step 2 examination history.*
Citizenship is as of the time of entrance into medical school.
Statistics for each examination are as of mailing date of examination results and do not include incompletes or those for whom scores were withheld.

Applicants who passed the former ECFMG English Test on or before March 3, 1999, have satisfied this requirement. Applicants who have not passed this test can satisfy the requirement by achieving a score acceptable to ECFMG on the Test of English as a Foreign Language (TOEFL). These applicants may take either a computer-based administration or a paper-based, Friday or Saturday (formerly special or international) administration of the TOEFL. Applicants who have never taken the ECFMG English Test must pass the TOEFL on or after March 4, 1999, to satisfy this requirement.

The TOEFL is offered throughout the world by the Educational Testing Service (ETS). For information and application materials for the TOEFL, contact:

Educational Testing Service
Princeton, NJ 08541
609 771-7100
E-mail: toefl@ets.org
www.toefl.org

Applicants who take the TOEFL to fulfill the English language proficiency requirement should refer to *Test of English as a Foreign Language (TOEFL)* in the ECFMG *Information Booklet* for information on the minimum score that the ECFMG will accept and instructions on how to have the ECFMG evaluate their TOEFL score.

Clinical Skills Assessment

The Clinical Skills Assessment (CSA) evaluates an examinee's ability to gather and interpret clinical patient data and communicate effectively in English. The CSA consists of eleven testing stations, ten of which are scored; in each station examinees encounter a Standardized Patient (SP), a lay person trained to realistically and consistently portray a patient. The SPs respond to questions from examinees with answers appropriate to the patient being portrayed and react appropriately to physical maneuvers. Examinees are expected to proceed through each encounter with an SP as they would with a real patient.

The CSA assesses whether an examinee can obtain a relevant medical history, perform a focused physical examination, and compose a written record of the patient encounter. The CSA also requires examinees to demonstrate proficiency in *spoken* English and appropriate interpersonal skills, as evaluated by the Standardized Patients encountered in the test stations.

Summary of Results of the Examination Program in 1999

In 1999, the USMLE was converted from paper and pencil administration to computer-based administration. The last paper and pencil administration of Step 2 was held on March 2-3, 1999. The ECFMG English Test was administered for the last time on March 3, 1999. Table 19 shows the results of these exams. There were no paper and pencil administrations of Step 1 in 1999.

Computer-based administrations of Step 1 and Step 2 began in May 1999 and August 1999, respectively. It is anticipated that the results of computer-based administrations of Step 1 and Step 2 in 1999 will be available for publication during the second half of 2000.

Standard ECFMG Certificates Issued in 1999

During 1999, 5,653 Standard ECFMG Certificates were issued. Table 20 shows the distribution of recipients of Standard ECFMG Certificates by country of medical school and citizenship. In 1999, medical schools in India and Dominica had the largest number of recipients: 979 (17.3%) were graduates of Indian medical schools and 363 (6.4%) of the recipients received their medical degrees in Dominica.

Based upon country of citizenship, citizens of the United States formed the largest group of recipients. Of the certificates issued in 1999, 1,233 (21.8%) were to US citizens. Citizens of India were the second largest group with 966 (17.1%) recipients.

Table 20

Standard ECFMG Certificates Issued in 1999: Distribution of Recipients by Country of Medical School and Citizenship

Country	Country of Medical School		Country of Citizenship	
	Number	%*	Number	%*
Australia	63	1.1	50	.9
Brazil	58	1.0	56	1.0
Canada	0	.0	67	1.2
China	208	3.7	207	3.7
Colombia	78	1.4	76	1.3
Dominica	363	6.4	5	.1
Dominican Republic	100	1.8	23	.4
Egypt	140	2.5	137	2.4
Germany	216	3.8	170	3.0
Grenada	352	6.2	3	.1
India	979	17.3	966	17.1
Iran	113	2.0	163	2.9
Ireland	63	1.1	38	.7
Israel	161	2.8	90	1.6
Italy	52	.9	39	.7
Lebanon	75	1.3	86	1.5
Mexico	78	1.4	43	.8
Montserrat	177	3.1	0	.0
Netherlands Antilles	80	1.4	0	.0
Nigeria	125	2.2	127	2.2
Pakistan	252	4.5	253	4.5
Philippines	166	2.9	111	2.0
Poland	74	1.3	53	.9
Romania	102	1.8	94	1.7
Russia	128	2.3	59	1.0
Syria	86	1.5	85	1.5
Turkey	72	1.3	68	1.2
United Kingdom	71	1.3	71	1.3
USA	0	.0	1,233	21.8
USSR*	0	.0	122	2.2
Countries with fewer than 50 recipients in both categories	1,134	9.6	1,019	8.6
Total for 1999	5,653	100	5,653	100

* The countries of the former USSR are represented separately.

Electronic Residency Application Service (ERAS)

Most residency programs require applicants to apply through the Electronic Residency Application Service (ERAS), which was developed by the Association of American Medical Colleges. ERAS transmits residency applications and supporting documents to residency program directors over the Internet. The ECFMG serves as the designated Dean's Office for students and graduates of foreign medical schools applying to residency programs through ERAS.

Specialties utilizing ERAS 2001 (for residency positions beginning in July 2001) are:

- Anesthesiology
- Dermatology
- Diagnostic Radiology
- Emergency Medicine
- Family Practice
- Family Practice/Physical Medicine and Rehabilitation combined programs
- Internal Medicine (Preliminary and Categorical)
- Internal Medicine/Emergency Medicine combined programs
- Internal Medicine/Family Practice combined programs
- Internal Medicine/Pediatrics combined programs
- Internal Medicine/Physical Medicine and Rehabilitation combined programs
- Internal Medicine/Psychiatry combined programs
- Obstetrics/Gynecology
- Orthopedic Surgery
- Pathology
- Pediatrics
- Pediatrics/Emergency Medicine combined programs
- Pediatrics/ Physical Medicine and Rehabilitation combined programs
- Physical Medicine and Rehabilitation
- Psychiatry
- Surgery
- Transitional Year
- All US Army and Navy programs

Additional specialties are expected to use ERAS for residency programs beginning in July 2002. Information on participating specialties for ERAS 2002 will be posted on the ERAS home page of the ECFMG web site as it becomes available. Applicants should contact residency program directors for specific requirements and deadlines.

To obtain an ERAS application materials request form and specific information on ERAS, applicants should visit the ECFMG web site at www.ecfmg.org. Applicants may also contact:

ECFMG ERAS Program
PO Box 13467
Philadelphia, PA 19101-3467
E-mail: erashelp@ecfmg.org
215 386-5900
215 222-5641 Fax

Visas

To obtain a visa to enter the United States to perform services as members of the medical profession or to receive graduate medical education, certain alien physicians are required, under the provisions of Public Law 94-484, to pass NBME Part I and Part II examinations or an examination determined to be equivalent for this purpose. The Secretary of Health and Human Services has recognized USMLE Step 1 and Step 2 as well as the former Visa Qualifying Examination (VQE) and the Foreign Medical Graduate Examination in the Medical Sciences (FMGEMS) as equivalent to NBME Part I and Part II examinations for the purposes of PL 94-484. To obtain additional information on visa requirements, foreign national physicians should refer to the Exchange Visitor Sponsorship Program home page of the ECFMG web site at www.ecfmg.org, US Embassies or Consulates abroad, or the US Immigration and Naturalization Service.

Table 21
Exchange Visitor Sponsorship Program for Physicians:
Number of J-1 Physicians in Graduate Medical Education
Programs in the United States, July 1, 1998, to June 30, 1999

Specialty	Count
Allergy and Immunology	57
Anesthesiology	649
Colon and Rectal Surgery	15
Dermatology	15
Diagnostic Radiology	269
Emergency Medicine	28
Family Practice	169
Internal Medicine	5,081
Internal Medicine/Emergency Medicine	2
Internal Medicine/Neurology	5
Internal Medicine/Pediatrics	51
Internal Medicine/Physical Medicine and Rehabilitation	1
Internal Medicine/Psychiatry	6
Medical Genetics	17
Neurology	467
Neurological Surgery	52
Nuclear Medicine	17
Obstetrics and Gynecology	96
Ophthalmology	100
Orthopedic Surgery	69
Otolaryngology	22
Pathology	343
Pediatrics	1,240
Pediatrics/Physical Medicine and Rehabilitation	2
Pediatrics/Psychiatry/Child Psychiatry	3
Physical Medicine and Rehabilitation	66
Plastic Surgery	36
Preventive Medicine	11
Psychiatry	732
Radiation Oncology	28
Surgery	490
Thoracic Surgery	89
Transitional Year	61
Urology	41
Total	**10,330**

Exchange Visitor Sponsorship Program

The ECFMG is authorized by the United States Department of State (DOS) to sponsor foreign national physicians as J-1 Exchange Visitors in ACGME-accredited graduate medical education programs. The objectives of this program are to enhance international exchange in the field of medicine and to promote mutual understanding between the people of the United States and other countries through the interchange of persons, knowledge, and skills.

The program is administered by ECFMG in accordance with the provisions set forth in an agreement between ECFMG and the DOS and the federal regulations established to implement the Mutual Educational and Cultural Exchange Act. ECFMG is responsible for ensuring that all Exchange Visitor Physicians and host institutions comply with the federal requirements for participation. ECFMG issues a Certificate of Eligibility for Exchange Visitor J-1 Status (Form IAP-66) for qualified applicants. This document must be processed through the United States Embassy or Consulate and the Immigration and Naturalization Service (INS) to secure the J-1 visa.

The Federal regulations refer to Exchange Visitor Physicians seeking J-1 sponsorship in accredited clinical programs as *alien physicians*. These applicants must meet the following general requirements:

- Pass USMLE Step 1 and Step 2 or the former VQE, NBME Part I and Part II, or FMGEMS (Note: The former 1-day ECFMG Examination does not meet the requirements for J-1 visa sponsorship.);

- Hold a valid Standard ECFMG Certificate (Graduates of LCME-accredited US and Canadian medical schools are not required to be ECFMG-certified.);

- Hold a contract or an official letter of offer for a position in an ACGME-accredited graduation medical education program that is affiliated with a medical school;

- Provide a statement of need from the Ministry of Health of the country of nationality or last legal permanent residence. This statement must provide written assurance that the country needs specialists in the area in which the Exchange Visitor will receive training and that he/she will return to the country upon completion.

(*Note:* If permanent residence is in a country other than that of citizenship, the Ministry of Health letter must come from the country of last legal permanent residence.)

The duration of stay for a J-1 Exchange Visitor Physician is limited to the time typically required to complete the advanced medical education program. This refers to the specialty and subspecialty certification requirements published by the American Board of Medical Specialties (ABMS). Participation is further limited to 7 years and is reserved for those progressing in accredited training programs.

J-1 Exchange Visitor Physicians sponsored for participation in nonclinical programs primarily involved with observation, consultation, teaching, or research are categorized as research scholars. Unlike alien physicians, participants in these programs generally do not have to pass US medical licensing or English examinations and are not required to be ECFMG-certified. Research scholars are limited to activities involving no patient contact or only incidental patient contact. The maximum period of participation for research scholars is 3 years.

Table 21 shows that the ECFMG sponsored 10,330 Exchange Visitor Physicians in US graduate medical education programs for the academic year July 1, 1998, to June 30, 1999. In the alien physician category, the ECFMG sponsored 6,285 in clinical residency (specialty) programs and 3,956 in clinical fellowships (subspecialty training) in 1998-1999. A total of 89 foreign nationals were sponsored in the research scholar category. Consistent with past trends, foreign nationals from India, Pakistan, and the Philippines represented a major segment (39%) of ECFMG-sponsored J-1 physicians for this period.

For application materials and specific information on ECFMG sponsorship, applicants should visit the ECFMG web site at www.ecfmg.org. Applicants may also contact:

Educational Commission for Foreign Medical Graduates
Exchange Visitor Sponsorship Program
3624 Market St
PO Box 41673
Philadelphia, PA 19101-1673
215 823-2121
215 386-9766 Fax

Certification Verification Service (CVS)

The ECFMG's Certification Verification Service provides primary source confirmation of the ECFMG certification status of graduates of foreign medical schools. The Joint Commission on Accreditation of Healthcare Organizations (JCAHO) has determined that an accredited health organization will satisfy the Joint Commission requirement for primary source verification of medical school completion for graduates of foreign medical schools if it confirms directly with the ECFMG that an applicant possesses a valid Standard ECFMG Certificate.

The ECFMG will confirm an applicant's certification status when a request is received in writing from a medical licensing authority, residency program director, hospital, or other organization that, in the judgment of ECFMG, has a legitimate interest in such information. Please note that there may be a fee for this service.

Requests for confirmation must contain the applicant's name, date of birth, and USMLE / ECFMG Identification Number, as well as the name and address of the organization to which the confirmation should be sent. Confirmations are mailed to the requesting organization within approximately 2 weeks. Confirmations are not sent to applicants directly.

For individuals who apply to residency programs through ERAS, the ECFMG automatically sends an electronic ECFMG status report at the time that their applications are processed to all of the programs to which they applied. If an applicant's ECFMG certification status changes during the ERAS application process, the ECFMG will automatically send an updated status report to all programs to which the applicant applied.

To obtain the appropriate request form(s) and additional information, refer to the CVS home page on the ECFMG web site at www.ecfmg.org or contact:

Educational Commission for Foreign Medical Graduates
CVS Department
PO Box 13679
Philadelphia PA 19101-3679
215 823-2115

Contact Information

The ECFMG Information Booklet, application materials for USMLE Step 1 and Step 2 and the ECFMG Clinical Skills Assessment, and general information on ECFMG certification are available on the ECFMG web site at www.ecfmg.org.

Individuals who do not have access to the Internet may request a copy of the ECFMG Information Booklet and application materials by calling (24 hours a day, 7 days a week):

- 800 500-8249, toll-free, from within North America, or
- 215 375-1913, from any location worldwide.

For requests by fax or mail or for specific inquiries, contact the ECFMG at:

ECFMG
3624 Market St
Philadelphia, PA 19104-2685
215 386-5900
215 387-9963 Fax

Immigration Overview for International Medical Graduates

Robert D. Aronson is a partner in the immigration law firm of Ingber & Aronson, which practices exclusively in the area of immigration and nationality law. The major area of his practice deals with immigration matters for foreign physicians and US medical institutions nationwide. He is the Chair of the Physicians Task Force of the American Immigration Lawyers Association and Vice Chair of the Association's Liaison Committee with the US Information Agency; he has also served as immigration consultant to the Commission on Graduate Medical Education (COGME).

This article outlines current immigration laws and policies that affect the physician community. This particular area of the law has become extremely complex owing to the continuing rapid changes within both the immigration and medical reform movements. In addition, a number of new laws and directives create various new opportunities as well as pitfalls to the immigration process for international medical graduates (IMGs) and their employing institutions.

Immigration Law Overview

All foreign nationals enter the United States in one of two broad immigration categories—either under a temporary, nonimmigrant visa or as a permanent resident. There are comparative advantages to both these categories. In the case of the temporary, nonimmigrant visa classifications, it is usually possible to gain this type of immigration coverage in a relatively short period of time. The two most common temporary, nonimmigrant classifications used by IMGs are the J-1 Exchange Visitor program and the H-1B temporary worker classification. However, both these classifications limit a physician's duration of residence in the United States and impose strict controls over the range of employment authorization, although they do have the advantage of being relatively quick to obtain. In contrast, permanent residence provides a foreign national with both an unlimited duration of residence and full, unrestricted employment authorization, although the processing time is much greater.

Temporary, Nonimmigrant Classifications

Most IMGs in graduate medical education (GME) programs arrive under the J-1 Exchange Visitor program. This program is administered by the US Information Agency (USIA) and is intended to provide a broad range of foreign nationals with educational, employment, and training opportunities in the United States.

An IMG applying for a J-1 visa must first obtain certification from the Educational Commission on Foreign Medical Graduates (ECFMG), the implementing agency for the J-1 Exchange Visitor program for physicians. To earn an ECFMG Certificate, an IMG must

1. pass stipulated examinations so as to establish medical competence, which at present consists solely of the United States Medical Licensing Examination (USMLE), Steps 1 and 2;

2. pass the ECFMG English language examination to establish English language competence;

3. possess an MD from a foreign medical school listed in the *World Directory of Medical Schools*, published by the World Health Organization.

All J-1 trainees must receive ECFMG Certification (Canadian medical school graduates are exempt from this requirement, because Canadian medical education and training are accredited under US standards).

Upon entry to the United States, an IMG is authorized to pursue GME for a period of up to 7 years to achieve stipulated training objectives. Each year, the GME program, in conjunction with the IMG, needs to file an extension application with the ECFMG.

Without exception, all J-1 physicians in clinical training are subject to a mandatory 2-year home residence obligation, regardless of country of citizenship or last permanent residence. In order for an IMG to ultimately qualify for permanent residence, he/she needs to either return to his/her home country for a 2-year period or obtain a waiver of this 2-year obligation.

By law, a waiver of this obligation is available only on the basis of the following three grounds:

- if the J-1 physician will suffer from persecution in his/her home country or country of last permanent residence;

- if fulfillment of the 2-year home residence obligation will subject a US citizen spouse or child to exceptional hardship; or

- based upon a recommendation issued by a government agency interested in the physician's continued residence/employment in the United States.

Without question, the vast majority of J-1 physicians who receive waivers do so on the basis of recommendations issued by government agencies. Generally speaking, such waivers fall within four basic patterns:

- employment by a federal agency, such as the Department of Veterans Affairs;

- recognition of outstanding academic and research achievements, as determined by the Department of Health and Human Services;

- service to medically underserved patient populations, particularly in rural communities, thereby falling within the interest of the US Department of Agriculture;

- pursuant to the sponsorship of a state Department of Health, under recent legislation that authorizes each state to sponsor up to 20 IMGs per year for waivers of their home residence obligation.

Rather than using the J-1 Exchange Visitor program, with its 2-year home residence requirement, an increasing number of foreign physicians are entering the United States under the H-1B Temporary Worker provisions. This visa classification enables a foreign national to enter the United States to accept professional-level employment for a period of up to 6 years. In most instances, H-1B coverage can be obtained within roughly 45 to 60 days.

In order for an IMG to qualify for H-1B benefits, all of the following four criteria must be met:

- possession of a full, unrestricted state medical license or the "appropriate authorization" for the position;

- an MD degree or a full unrestricted foreign license;

- English language competence as established either through graduation from an accredited medical school or by passing the ECFMG English language exam;

- the Federation Licensing Examination (FLEX) or its equivalents—the National Board of Medical Examiners (NBME), Parts I, II, and III, or the USMLE, Steps 1, 2, and 3.

As a result of this FLEX equivalency issue, most Canadian physicians do not qualify for H-1B benefits. The standard Canadian medical credential—the Licentiate of the Medical Council of Canada (LMCC)—is widely accepted among the states for medical licensure. Therefore, most Canadian physicians have traditionally not had any reason to sit for the FLEX or its stipulated equivalents. In this manner, H-1B immigration requirements have established different credentialing standards from those of the state medical licensure boards, which have traditionally been the primary judge of physician competence.

Permanent Residence Strategies

There are various ways for a foreign national to qualify for permanent residence, ranging from familial relationships with US citizens or permanent residents to fear of persecution so as to merit refugee entitlement. In most instances, though, an IMG will need to qualify for permanent residence based upon an employment position. In a sense, there are four basic pathways to permanent residence based upon employment as a physician.

Pathway One—A highly attractive pathway to employment-based permanent residence is based upon National Interest Waiver criteria. In this instance, an IMG has a streamlined, expedited pathway to permanent residence if it can be shown that his/her employment as a physician carries potential major benefits to areas of high national interest. If this can be established, the immigration filing is made directly to the Immigration and Naturalization Service, thereby skipping over entirely the filing process to the Department of Labor, as described below. Within a clinical setting, this National Interest Waiver strategy has been used over the years to facilitate the relocation of physicians to designated medically underserved areas.

The National Interest Waiver approach for physicians was terminated for a period of time owing to an administrative decision in August 1998. In November 1999, however, Congress restored the National Interest Waiver eligibility for physicians working either within designated medically underserved areas and/or within Veterans Affairs facilities. Any physician applying for this streamlined immigration procedure needs to fulfill a 5-year period of service working specifically within a medically underserved area and/or a VA facility to gain eligibility to actually receive permanent resident status.

Pathway Two—A second employment-based pathway to permanent residence involves a three-step process. The first and arguably most complex stage is the Labor Certification Application process. Conducted under the auspices of the US Department of Labor, this procedure establishes that employing a foreign national/IMG will not harm the US labor market, particularly by taking a job away from a fully qualified US worker. Therefore, acting under a complex recruitment/advertisement procedure, the employer needs to show that the IMG is not simply the most qualified applicant but is rather the only fully qualified candidate for the specific employment position.

After completing the Labor Certification Application process, the employer must submit an Immigrant Visa Petition to the Immigration and Naturalization Service (INS), establishing the complete suitability of the IMG for the position. Upon approval of this petition, the IMG is able to actually apply for permanent residence either through an INS District Office (adjustment of status) or through a US Consular post (consular processing).

Note: An IMG needs to possess either an ECFMG certificate or an MD from an Liaison Committee for Medical Education (LCME)-accredited medical school (ie, generally US or Canadian). Also, an IMG cannot finalize the application for permanent residence status if he/she has an unfulfilled or unwaived J-1 2-year home residence obligation.

Pathway Three—A variant on the process above enables an employer to request a waiver of any further recruiting/advertising obligations. Such waivers are granted by the US Department of Labor when the employer has fully and in good faith recruited within the previous 6-month period, through which it legitimately came to the conclusion that there are no fully qualified US applicants for the open position.

Pathway Four—A final option to permanent residence is available to physicians of extraordinarily high professional capabilities, working either in clinical practice or in academic medicine. Such individuals may qualify for permanent residence under an expedited procedure established either for Aliens of Extraordinary Ability or Outstanding Professors or Researchers.

New Legal Developments

A major new piece of legislation has extended the State 20 Waiver program for a 6-year period, through June 1, 2002. This program empowers each state to recommend waivers for up to 20 IMGs per year, provided that they work in a designated medically underserved area for at least 3 years. At present, roughly 38 states have implemented their own waiver program.

Many IMGs, particularly from third world countries, have traditionally processed for their visas through US Consulates in the neighboring countries of Canada or Mexico. The new law creates certain major new restrictions on visa processing in Canada or Mexico, although some concessions have been granted to physicians who intend to work in designated medically underserved communities.

One new law cuts down considerably on instances in which the humanitarian benefits of a physician's services to a medically underserved area can be considered for the interim issuance of an employment authorization document.

Another new law has also created major new bars to permanent residence for foreign nationals who have resided illegally within the United States for extended periods of time. This provision is certainly not targeted directly at physicians, but is rather an across-the-board provision intended to create a major new disincentive for violating US immigration laws.

The most wide ranging legislative initiative of note involves the restoration of National Interest Waiver entitlement to physicians working within designated medically underserved areas and/or VA facilities. As noted above, permanent residence based upon the filing of a National Interest Waiver obligates the physician to fulfill a 5-year period of employment in a designated medically underserved area and/or a VA facility prior to gaining eligibility for permanent resident status. The purpose of this legislative initiative is to facilitate the relocation of physicians into employment positions which have traditionally been underserved by the domestic physician workforce.

Section IV.

Federal and National Programs and Activities

Licensure in the US Armed Forces

Department of the Air Force

Gary H. Murray, Brigadier General,USAF, DC
Commander, Air Force Medical Operations Agency
Sharon R. Ahrari, Lieutenant Colonel, USAF, NC
Deputy Chief, Clinical Performance Improvement
Office of the Surgeon General
Washington, DC

The Department of the Air Force's licensure policy is consistent with that of the Department of Defense (DOD). Air Force physicians must possess a current, valid, unrestricted license. The license must be from an official agency of a state; the District of Columbia; or a commonwealth, territory, or possession of the United States to provide health care independently within the scope of the license.

These licensure requirements apply to both military and DOD health care personnel employed by the Air Force. DOD health care personnel shall be required to have taken and passed a licensure or otherwise authorizing examination at the time an individual completes all didactic and clinical requirements and is eligible for the first time to take the necessary examinations. Before examination and receipt of the license or other authorizing document, clinical practice will be limited to practice under supervision.

Civilian health care personnel considering employment or other affiliation with the DOD health care system who have trained through civilian schools or programs and who have had the opportunity to test for licensure or other authorizing document must possess and maintain a current, valid, and unrestricted license or other authorizing document before direct accession or other affiliation with the DOD.

Department of the Army

Sid W. Atkinson, MD, Colonel
Director, Quality Management
US Army Medical Command
Ft. Sam Houston, Texas

The Clinical Standards Division within the Department of the Army Medical Command is responsible for developing policy and overseeing all facets of quality improvement, credentials review and privileging, licensure, and risk management for the Army Surgeon General. The Division acts as the working information office concerning clinical standards issues and accreditation by the Joint Commission for Accreditation of Healthcare Organizations for US Army medicine worldwide.

Department of Defense physicians (military and civilian, civilian contract, and partnership) must possess a current, valid, unrestricted license from an official agency of a state; the District of Columbia; or a commonwealth, territory, or possession of the United States to provide health care independently within the scope of their licenses. Physicians in graduate medical education (GME) programs must possess a license within 1 year from the completion of their first year of GME training. An exception exists for individuals who complete their first year of GME in a state requiring 2 or more years of GME for licensure and who are assigned within that same state in continuity. These individuals must possess a license within 1 year of completion of their second year of GME training. Licenses issued by authorities allowing reduced or no fees for military personnel will be considered valid if the issuing authority accepts and considers current information in determining continued licensure. Health care providers with pending required license or certification may work only under the supervision of a licensed provider of the same or a similar professional discipline.

Department of the Navy

John Chandler, Commander, Medical Corps, US Navy
Clinical Management and Plans Division
Bureau of Medicine and Surgery
Department of the Navy
Washington, DC

Georgi Irvine, Commander, Nurse Corps, US Navy
Service Line Manager, Medical and Dental Staff Services
Naval Healthcare Support Office
Jacksonville, Florida

The Clinical Management and Plans Division within the Bureau of Medicine and Surgery, Department of the Navy (DON), is responsible for developing policy and directing the development and implementation of US Navy-wide quality management and professional affairs programs to improve the quality of patient care; reduce risks to our customers, guests, and staff; advance good stewardship; and maintain accreditation by the Joint Commission for Accreditation of Healthcare Organizations of all US Navy fixed medical treatment facilities.

Federal regulations require physicians and other health providers within the military health services system to possess a professional license or certification. The DON further requires the license to be current, valid, unrestricted, and one to which quality management data accrues. All DON physicians (military, civilian, civilian contract, and partnership), except interns, must possess a license from a recognized, official agency of a state; the District of Columbia; or a commonwealth, territory, or possession of the United States to provide health care services independently within the scope of their license. Licenses issued by authorities allowing reduced or no fees for military personnel must meet the same licensure criteria. Health care practitioners lacking required license or certification may work only under a plan of supervision with a licensed practitioner of the same or a similar professional discipline. This policy supports the US Navy's goal to ensure all practitioners are available for worldwide assignment and rapid deployment.

Federal Controlled Substances Registration

Office of Diversion Control
Drug Enforcement Administration
Washington, DC

Provisions of the Controlled Substances Act of 1970 (CSA) mandate that pharmaceuticals falling under its authority be maintained in a "closed system of distribution" that oversees all phases of manufacture, distribution, and dispensing. The Department of Justice, through the Drug Enforcement Administration (DEA), is entrusted with devising and administering a program that ensures the availability of controlled substances for the ultimate user, the patient, while preventing their diversion into illicit markets.

The backbone of the DEA's efforts is the controlled substances registration program. This program, through its implementing regulations, requires that any person desiring to manufacture, distribute, or dispense controlled substances must register with the DEA. After approval, each applicant is assigned a unique registration number, which must be used in every transaction involving controlled substances. Use of the DEA registration number, together with required records of transactions, allows tracking of controlled substances from the point of manufacture to the point at which they are dispensed to the patient.

As of April 4, 2000, there were 1,017,449 active DEA registrants. Medical practitioners account for 884,789 of those registrants, with an additional 60,000 new applications for registration received each year.

Applying for registration as a medical practitioner is a relatively simple process. A physician who seeks to become registered with the DEA must submit an application on DEA Form 224 together with the required fee to:

Drug Enforcement Administration
Registration Unit
PO Box 28083, Central Station
Washington, DC 20005

800 882-9539
www.deadiversion.usdoj.gov

The form can be obtained from the Registration Unit or any DEA field office with a registration assistant.

Following initial processing by the Registration Unit, the application is referred to the appropriate DEA field office for a records check and verification with state licensing authorities that the practitioner is properly licensed and authorized by the state to handle controlled substances. Barring any problems, the registration is then approved and a certificate bearing the practitioner's DEA registration number is issued. This process normally takes from 4 to 6 weeks to complete. (Renewal applications generally are processed within 2 weeks). The DEA certificate must be maintained at the registered location and must be kept available for official inspection.

Under special circumstances, applications may be faxed, but the completed forms cannot be returned for processing via facsimile. Completed applications must be mailed with the appropriate fee and an original signature. Completed application packages may be sent via overnight delivery, but the DEA will not incur the cost of any delivery service. Due to security requirements, all parcels received by the DEA are scanned in an off-site location prior to delivery. This requirement will add 1 day to the time it takes to receive packages. Non-US Postal Service deliveries should be addressed to:

Drug Enforcement Administration
attn: Registration Unit, ODRR
2401 Jefferson Davis Highway
Alexandria, VA 22301

The DEA also registers mid-level practitioners (MLPs) who have been authorized by the appropriate state licensing agency to handle controlled substances. Currently over 46,000 MLPs, including nurse practitioners, certified nurse-midwives, physician assistants, and optometrists, are registered with the DEA. MLPs apply for registration on the same application forms as other practitioners. MLP registration numbers begin with the letter "M" rather than the letters "A" or "B," which are issued to other practitioners.

The fee for both new and renewal applications for all practitioners is $210 for a 3-year period. The exemption from payment of the application fee is limited to federal, state, or local government-operated hospitals or institutions.

A practitioner's registration must be renewed every 3 years. Each practitioner is issued a renewal application, DEA Form 224a, approximately 45 days before the expiration date of his or her registration. Registrants who do not receive the form can contact any local DEA office with a registration assistant. DEA registrations are issued for controlled substances activities at specific locations. If a physician has more than one office at which controlled substances will be administered and/or dispensed, a separate registration must be obtained for each location. However, this requirement applies only to those locations away from the principal location at which controlled substances will be administered or dispensed. If the activities at secondary locations are restricted to prescribing only, then separate registration is not required.

When dealing with the DEA on registration issues, practitioners should be aware of the following:

1. When filing a new or renewal application, or requesting modification of a registration, file early; DEA's registration program receives over 400,000 filings per year.

2. One of the primary criteria for issuing a DEA registration is that the applicant be authorized by the state in which he or she will practice. Make sure that all necessary applications, etc, for state licensing have been taken care of before filing your application for DEA registration. The same applies for registrants relocating from one state to another.

3. Keep track of your registration expiration date. Between 20,000 and 30,000 renewal notices are mailed to registrants each month. There is no guarantee that all of them will be received by the registrants. If a registration does expire, that registration cannot be used for any purpose, and the registrant is no longer authorized to handle controlled substances. Until the registration is renewed and a new certificate of registration is issued, use of the registration is a violation of the law.

4. As noted earlier, DEA registrations are issued for controlled substances activities at a specific location. Therefore, the Registration Unit or appropriate DEA field office must be notified in advance of any change of address. Further, the registration address cannot be a post office box but the actual location at which controlled substances activities take place. If there are problems with postal delivery or the address that should be used, contact the Registration Unit or local DEA office before filing.

5. The Registration Unit can be contacted toll-free at

   800 882-9539

   Whenever contacting the DEA regarding an existing registration, reference the DEA registration number. Further, if the matter is considered important, conduct it in writing. During busy periods, the Registration Unit receives thousands of calls each week; a mental note is easier to lose than a letter.

The DEA's registration program plays an extremely important role in efforts to control the diversion of legitimately produced controlled substances to the illicit market. The program has grown in complexity with the addition of new substances, such as anabolic steroids, and a new category of registration—mid-level practitioners—for advanced practice nurses, certified nurse midwives, physician assistants, and others. The continued success of the program is the result of the combined efforts and understanding of health care professionals, industry, and the DEA.

National Practitioner Data Bank

The National Practitioner Data Bank collects and releases information on physicians' medical malpractice payments, adverse licensure actions, adverse clinical privilege actions, adverse professional society membership actions, and exclusions from participation in Medicare and Medicaid. Responsibility for its implementation resides in the Division of Quality Assurance, Bureau of Health Professions, US Department of Health and Human Services (HHS). Signed into law in 1986, the Data Bank began collecting and disseminating information in 1990.

The Data Bank is an alert or flagging system to facilitate a comprehensive review of health care practitioners' professional credentials—licensure, professional society memberships, medical malpractice payment history, and record of clinical privileges. Hospitals, professional societies, and state licensing boards use the Data Bank's information, in conjunction with information from other sources, when granting clinical privileges or in employment, affiliation, or licensure decisions. State medical boards must report certain adverse licensure actions related to professional competence or professional conduct and any changes to such actions. Hospitals, professional societies, and other health care organizations are also required to report certain data to the Data Bank.

Data Availability and Confidentiality

Information reported to the Data Bank is considered confidential and is available only to state licensing boards; hospitals and other health care entities, including professional societies; and others as specified in the law. Information is not available to the general public.

Practitioners are allowed to query their own records in the Data Bank at any time; the fee for self-queries is $10. If a practitioner has been the subject of an Adverse Action Report or Medical Malpractice Payment Report submitted to the Data Bank, a list of all parties to whom the reported information has been disclosed will be included with the response.

Reporting

After processing a report from a reporting entity, the Data Bank sends a notice to the entity and to the subject practitioner. In the event of errors, practitioners must contact the reporting entity to request that it correct the information. The Data Bank is prohibited by law from modifying information submitted in reports.

A practitioner who is the subject of a Data Bank report may add a statement to the report, dispute either the factual accuracy of the information in a report or whether the report was submitted in accordance with Data Bank reporting requirements, or both.

Responsibilities of State Medical Boards

State medical boards must report certain disciplinary actions related to professional competence or conduct taken against physicians' licenses. These actions include revocation, suspension, censure, reprimand, probation, and surrender. Boards must also report revisions to adverse licensure actions. Any board that fails to comply with Data Bank reporting requirements can have its reporting responsibility removed by the Secretary of HHS. In these cases, the Secretary will designate another qualified entity to report Data Bank information.

Available Materials

Materials available from the Data Bank include the *National Practitioner Data Bank Guidebook*; entity registration materials; *QPRAC, A Guide for Users*; fact sheets on various topics; and practitioner self-query materials.

National Practitioner Data Bank
PO Box 10832, Chantilly, VA 20151
800 767-6732
www.npdb-hipdb.com

Section V.

Other Organizations and Programs

American Board of Medical Specialties

The American Board of Medical Specialties (ABMS) is a nonprofit organization of 24 approved medical specialty boards. These 24 boards (listed below) have been approved by the ABMS and the AMA Council on Medical Education (AMA CME) through the Liaison Committee for Specialty Boards (LCSB), with ultimate approval of the application by the membership of the ABMS and the AMA CME.

American Board of:

- Allergy and Immunology
- Anesthesiology
- Colon and Rectal Surgery
- Dermatology
- Emergency Medicine
- Family Practice
- Internal Medicine
- Medical Genetics
- Neurological Surgery
- Nuclear Medicine
- Obstetrics and Gynecology
- Ophthalmology
- Orthopaedic Surgery
- Otolaryngology
- Pathology
- Pediatrics
- Physical Medicine and Rehabilitation
- Plastic Surgery
- Preventive Medicine
- Psychiatry and Neurology
- Radiology
- Surgery
- Thoracic Surgery
- Urology

The mission of the ABMS is to maintain and improve the quality of medical care by helping its member boards develop and use professional and educational standards for the evaluation and certification of physician specialists. The certification of physicians provides assurance to the public that a physician specialist certified by an ABMS member board has successfully completed an approved educational program and an evaluation process that assesses the knowledge, skills, and experience required to provide quality patient care in that specialty. Medical specialty board certification is an additional process to receiving a medical degree, completing residency training, and receiving a license to practice medicine.

In collaboration with the other organizations and agencies concerned, the approved medical specialty boards assist in improving the quality of medical education by elevating the standards of graduate medical education and approving facilities for specialty training.

The actual accreditation review for the approval of residency programs in each specialty is conducted by a Residency Review Committee on which the respective specialty board has equal representation with the AMA Council on Medical Education and, in some cases, with a related specialty society.

For more information about the ABMS, its member boards, and the process of developing and using standards for the evaluation and certification of physician specialists, contact:

American Board of Medical Specialties
1007 Church St/Ste 404
Evanston, IL 60201-5913
847 491-9091
847 328-3596 Fax
www.abms.org

Medical Specialty Board Certification and its Relationship to Licensure

Stephen H. Miller, MD, MPH
Executive Vice President
American Board of Medical Specialties
Evanston, Illinois

Arthur Osteen, PhD
Director
Department of PRA, Policy and Liaison Activities
American Medical Association
Chicago, Illinois

From its inception, medical specialty certification in the United States has been a voluntary process. Since the establishment of the first nationally recognized medical specialty board in 1917, some physicians have elected to seek formal recognition of their qualifications in their chosen specialty fields by presenting themselves for examination before specialty boards composed of their professional peers. The definitions of each of the specialties and of the educational and other requirements leading to eligibility for board certification have been developed by consensus within the medical profession. This process of certification of a medical specialist has remained separate and distinct from licensure by civil authorities of professionals qualified to practice medicine within their jurisdictions.

The American Board of Medical Specialties (ABMS) is the umbrella organization for the 24 medical specialty boards authorized and recognized to certify physician specialists in the United States. The 24 boards have been approved by the ABMS and the AMA Council on Medical Education (AMA CME) through the Liaison Committee for Specialty Boards (LCSB), with ultimate approval of the application by the membership of the ABMS and the AMA CME.

The primary function of the ABMS is to maintain and improve the quality of medical care by assisting the member boards in their efforts to develop and use standards for the evaluation and certification of physician specialists.

The intent of the certification process is to improve the quality of patient care by providing assurance to the public that a certified physician specialist has successfully completed an approved educational program and an evaluation, including an examination process designed to assess the knowledge, skills, and experience necessary for the provision of quality patient care in that specialty.

The ABMS Statement on "Relationship Between Specialty Board Certification and Medical Licensure"

The ABMS encourages its member boards to require unlimited medical licensure as a prerequisite for certification and maintenance of such licensure for recertification. This is one of several criteria the boards may use in satisfying themselves as to the moral character and legal standing of candidates in their respective states. A number of state licensing boards now accept certification by a specialty board in lieu of their own requirements for licensure.

Although the ABMS recognizes the right of each state to establish its own regulations, ABMS discourages the substitution of certification for licensure requirements because it has led in some cases to licensure by specialty. The ABMS opposes licensure by specialty for the following reasons:

1. It is convinced that every specialist should maintain basic knowledge and skill in the broad aspects of medical care.

2. The boundaries between specialties are often hazy and overlapping. State governments should not define such boundaries lest transgressions be punishable under the law. ABMS believes that practice restrictions should be determined only by the judgment of individual physicians, the medical staffs of hospitals, or the customs of the community in which the doctor practices.

3. Licensure by specialty will impose serious handicaps on physicians who seek interstate endorsement of licenses so obtained. Very few state licensing boards will endorse licenses obtained by specialty certification.

4. Requiring a physician to limit his or her practice to a specialty could increase the cost of medical care as it might entail needless consultations with unnecessary repetition of tests with concomitant increases in patients' bills.

Furthermore, the laws of many states either permit or require licensing boards to establish rules and regulations mandating continuing medical education (CME) for reregistration of medical licenses. Some state boards will accept specialty board recertification as satisfying their CME requirements.

Although the ABMS recognizes the right of each state to establish its own regulations, it discourages the acceptance of recertification in lieu of the state's reregistration requirements for the following reasons:

1. There is danger that this could encourage a trend toward licensure by specialty.

2. As recertification is private and voluntary, it is undesirable to adopt this as a substitute for the public and legal requirements of licensing boards.

Approved by the ABMS Assembly, January 28, 1977; reaffirmed on March 20, 1997.

Definition of "Board Eligible"

"Board eligible" is a term frequently used to describe a physician who has completed a period of specialty education but has not been specialty board-certified. Usually the term is understood to mean that the physician has completed the years of graduate medical education required for certification but has not taken the specialty board examination.

Official ABMS policy states that the term "board eligible" should not be used. Instead, physicians and medical organizations should state exactly what a physician's circumstances are in regard to certification. For example, physicians planning to seek or seeking board certification might state that they have completed the years of residency required for admission to the examination, have been admitted to the examination, or have passed the examination and will be provided with a certificate. Physicians who do not plan to seek board certification should specifically state their qualifications for practice, including any special training or honors.

AMA Policy Regarding Specialty Board Certification and Licensure

AMA policy, like that of the ABMS, opposes licensure by specialty. The earliest statement of this policy comes in a report of the AMA Council on Medical Education (CME): "Experience with licensure by specialty is too limited to determine what the long-range effects will be in the provision of timely, safe, and comprehensive medical care. However, the AMA does not consider licensure by specialty to be desirable even in unusual cases." This position was reaffirmed by a report of the Council on Long Range Planning and Development in 1990. Discussions in CME meetings indicate support for the position that all physicians, regardless of their specialties, should have knowledge of general medicine, that is, they should be able to identify illnesses and disorders and refer patients to other physicians if necessary. Licensure based on specialty education and specialty examinations would be insufficient to ensure that physicians have a broad base of general medical knowledge.

The AMA has also adopted a policy that hospitals and managed care organizations should be able to appoint to staff physicians who do not have specialty board certificates. The most recent statement of this policy is from AMA CME Report 5, adopted at the 1996 Interim Meeting: "[It is recommended that] the AMA reaffirm policy that decisions regarding staff appointment should be based upon the training, experience, and demonstrated competence of candidates and not exclusively upon the presence or absence of board certification; and that third party payers not exclude non-board certified physicians as a class from participation in their programs, without regard to individual training, experience, and current competence."

The AMA has communicated the policy to hospitals and to managed care organizations, many of which have physicians on staff who do not have specialty board certificates.

The AMA recognizes the importance of specialty board certification and supports the certification process. The AMA, for instance, is a member of the Liaison Committee on Specialty Boards, which has established procedures for the recognition of new boards that become members of the ABMS. The AMA also recognizes that there are competent physicians who do not have board certificates.

Accreditation Council for Graduate Medical Education

The Accreditation Council for Graduate Medical Education (ACGME) is an accrediting agency composed of directors nominated by five national associations interested in graduate medical education:

- American Board of Medical Specialties
- American Hospital Association
- American Medical Association
- Association of American Medical Colleges
- Council of Medical Specialty Societies.

The federal government names a representative to serve in a nonvoting capacity, and the ACGME chooses three public directors. There is also a resident director appointed by the Resident Physicians Section of the AMA, with the advice of other national organizations that represent residents, and the chair of the Residency Review Committee Council sits as a voting director.

A Residency Review Committee (RRC) consists of representatives appointed by the AMA, the appropriate specialty board, and, in some cases, a national specialty organization. The Transitional Year Review Committee is composed of nine members who are appointed by the chair of the ACGME in conjunction with the Executive Committee. The term "review committee" is used to denote a Residency Review Committee and the Transitional Year Review Committee.

GME programs are accredited either by the ACGME upon the recommendation of an appropriate review committee, or by the review committee itself, if accreditation authority has been delegated by the ACGME. Accreditation of a residency program indicates that it is judged to be in substantial compliance with the *Essentials of Accredited Residencies in Graduate Medical Education* (*Essentials*), which includes the Institutional Requirements and the relevant Program Requirements. The jurisdiction of the ACGME is limited to programs in the United States, its territories, and its possessions.

A list of programs accredited by the ACGME, including detailed information about each program, is published annually by the AMA in the *Graduate Medical Education Directory*. With the exception of that information, the contents of program files are confidential, as are all other documents regarding a program used by a review committee.

For more information, contact:

Accreditation Council for Graduate Medical Education
515 N State St, 20th Fl
Chicago, IL 60610
312 464-4920
312 464-4098 Fax
www.acgme.org

AMA Continuing Medical Education Programs and Activities

Physicians' participation in group and individual self-learning activities reflects a commitment to provide patients with the most appropriate treatments, services, and information. The American Medical Association (AMA) supports these physician efforts by:

- recognizing completion of CME;
- providing online information about accredited CME activities;
- offering CME publications and programs (online and enduring programs, monographs, and AMA conferences and courses); and
- conducting train-the-trainer programs.

The AMA Physician's Recognition Award

Established by the AMA House of Delegates in 1968, the AMA Physician's Recognition Award (PRA) encourages participation in CME and acknowledges the individual physician's participation in CME activities. About 20,000 physicians apply for the PRA each year; 60,000 have valid AMA PRA certificates. Activities that meet education standards established by the AMA can be designated "AMA PRA category 1" by educational institutions accredited to provide CME, such as state medical societies, medical specialty societies, medical schools, and hospitals. Other activities may be reported for category 2.

PRA certificates are provided in lengths of 1, 2, or 3 years; in addition, two types of certificates are available—the standard certificate and the certificate with commendation for self-directed learning (see Table 22).

Through reciprocity arrangements, the AMA will award the PRA certificate if the CME requirements of the following organizations are met:

- American Academy of Dermatology
- American Academy of Family Physicians
- American Academy of Ophthalmology
- American Academy of Otolaryngology – Head and Neck Surgery
- American Academy of Pediatrics
- American College of Obstetricians and Gynecologists
- American College of Emergency Physicians
- American College of Preventive Medicine
- American Psychiatric Association
- American Society of Anesthesiologists
- American Society of Clinical Pathologists/ College of American Pathologists

Table 22
AMA Physician's Recognition Award (PRA) Certificate Options and Requirements

Certificate	Type	Category 1 hours	Category 2 hours	Category 1 or 2 hours
1 year certificate–50 hours	Standard certificate	20		30
	Certificate with commendation	20	20	10
2 year certificate–100 hours	Standard certificate	40		60
	Certificate with commendation	40	40	20
3 year certificate–150 hours	Standard certificate	60		90
	Certificate with commendation	60	60	30

Note: *Reading is **not** reportable as category 2 for the certificate with commendation, but reading **is** reportable for the standard certificate. Applicants for either certificate must indicate that they have read medical literature an average of 2 hours per week.*

- American Society of Plastic and Reconstructive Surgeons
- American Urological Association
- California Medical Association
- Medical Society of New Jersey
- Medical Society of Virginia
- National Medical Association

The PRA is also accepted by a number of states as evidence that CME required for licensure reregistration has been completed. Participation in lectures and demonstration activities, as well as self-learning activities, can be reported.

The AMA sends PRA application forms to physicians who have had a valid PRA certificate within the past 3 years, physicians whose current certificate is expiring within 3 months, physicians in residency programs, and physicians who have completed a residency program within the last 5 years. The AMA PRA application form and instruction booklet are available at www.ama-assn.org/cme. They can also be obtained from:

PRA Department
Continuing Physician Professional Development
American Medical Association
515 N State St
Chicago, IL 60610
312 464-4669   312 464-4567 Fax

Online Information About Accredited CME Activities

The AMA Online CME Locator (www.ama-assn.org/cme) is a database of more than 2,000 category 1 activities for the AMA PRA. All listed sponsors are accredited by the Accreditation Council for Continuing Medical Education.

The Continuing Medical Education Resource Guide (www.ama-assn.org/cme) provides information on the many facets of CME planning and participation. It includes information on CME requirements, CME membership organizations and international CME conferences, ethics in CME, and telemedicine.

AMA CME Programs

R. Mark Evans, PhD
Dept. of Healthcare Education Products and Standards
American Medical Association

Enduring (Self-Assessment) CME Programs

The AMA Healthcare Education Products Group offers a number of enduring CME programs that provide physician self-assessment. These programs offer quality CME in a convenient format that permits learners to work at their own pace and at a time that fits a busy clinical schedule.

The Healthcare Education Products Group, which offers enduring CME programs in print, CD-ROM, and Internet formats, is dedicated to improving the effectiveness and scope of CME programs by exploring new formats and delivery approaches for CME programs that tap into the latest clinical information and that meet the AMA's rigorous CME standards.

Monographs

The AMA produces and distributes printed self-study monographs, which are developed in cooperation with medical specialty societies and recognized medical experts. These programs are intended for primary care physicians and other interested medical specialists. Monographs and patient education are available in the following areas:

Respiratory Disorders
- Managing Asthma Today (I): Integrating New Concepts (2 hours)
- Managing Asthma Today (II): Common Comorbidities and Select Patient Populations (2 hours)

Viral STDs
- Genital Herpes: A Clinician's Guide to Diagnosis and Treatment (4 hours)
- External Genital Warts: Diagnosis and Treatment (2 hours)

Neurological Conditions
- Managing Migraine Today (two parts) (4 hours)

Women's Health
- Managing Osteoporosis (three parts)
- Genetic Susceptibility Testing for Breast and Ovarian Cancer (2 hours)

Endocrine and Metabolic Disorders
- Managing Diabetes (two parts)

Disorders of the Immune System, Connective Tissue, and Joints
- Managing Osteoarthritis

Another example of an AMA monograph with AMA PRA category 1 hours is Medical Management of the Home Care Patient: Guidelines for Physicians, for which physicians may receive up to 3 hours of PRA category 1 credit.

Internet Programs

The AMA provides Web-based CME programs on such topics as osteoporosis, osteoarthritis, diabetes, migraine, and asthma. These convenient programs, based on the enduring CME monographs described above, are developed with the assistance of national experts and make use of nationally recognized clinical practice guidelines. These educational programs have been awarded AMA PRA category 1 hours.

Journal CME

Since 1997, the AMA has designated selected articles in the *Journal of the American Medical Association* Reader's Choice and the *Archives* journals for AMA PRA category 1 credit.

AMA-sponsored Conference and Live Events

As an accredited CME provider, the AMA sponsors multiple conferences and live events designated for category 1 credit. Participants receive education on various topics of interest to all disciplines and specialties.

International CME

Since 1996, the AMA has recognized the value of collaborating with organizations in other countries to sponsor international events offering CME. Interested organizations complete an application reviewed by the AMA to ensure that the content and format meet specified standards. American physicians attending these conferences may receive category 1 credit, with required documentation. For more information, contact Julie Johnston at 312 464-5196.

Information

For more information on AMA CME programs and activities in particular, contact

Multimedia CME	312 464-5990
AMA CME credits/courses	312 464-4952
CME Resource Guide	312 464-4637
Physician's Recognition Award	312 464-4669
Credentials/licensure	312 464-4677
International CME	312 464-5196

For general information, contact:

Continuing Physician Professional Development
American Medical Association
515 N State St
Chicago, IL 60610
312 464-4671
312 464-5830 Fax

Project USA: Opportunity to Travel and Serve

Primary care physicians with a full and unrestricted license are being sought to participate in Project USA. This American Medical Association program is designed to recruit physicians for temporary short-term replacement service at Indian Health Service hospitals and clinics in several western states to enable US Public Health Service physicians to take vacations or fulfill continuing education requirements. Openings are available year round for 2 to 4 (or more) weeks. These locum tenens positions provide a weekly salary, malpractice insurance coverage, and round trip coach airfare. Living accommodations are also available. For more information, contact John Naughton, American Medical Association, 312 464-4702.

Joint Commission on Accreditation of Healthcare Organizations

An independent, nonprofit organization, the Joint Commission on Accreditation of Healthcare Organizations (JCAHO), or Joint Commission, evaluates and accredits approximately 19,000 health care organizations and programs in the United States and other countries. Accreditation by the Joint Commission is nationally recognized as a symbol of quality indicating that an organization meets state-of-the-art performance standards.

Joint Commission staff work with health care experts, providers, researchers, purchasers, and consumers around the world to develop optimally achievable performance standards, all with a single focus—to improve the safety and quality of patient care.

To earn and maintain accreditation, organizations must undergo an on-site survey by a team of Joint Commission surveyors at least every 3 years (laboratories are surveyed every 2 years). The Joint Commission employs more than 700 experienced physicians, nurses, health care administrators, medical technologists, psychologists, pharmacists, and other medical professionals to conduct these surveys.

Accreditation Programs

The Joint Commission operates the eight accreditation programs, listed below, that serve various types of health care organizations:

- *Assisted Living Accreditation Program*
- *Hospital Accreditation Program*
- *Home Care Accreditation Program*
- *Ambulatory Care Accreditation Program*
- *Laboratory Accreditation Program*
- *Long Term Care Accreditation Program*
- *Behavioral Health Care Accreditation Program*
- *Network Accreditation Program*

Benefits of Accreditation

Accreditation by the Joint Commission

- assists organizations in improving the safety and quality of the care they provide;
- strengthens community confidence;
- provides professional consultation and ongoing support;
- enhances staff education and recruitment;
- fulfills licensure requirements in many states;
- attracts professional referrals;
- may convey Medicare and Medicaid certification; and
- is recognized by insurers, expedites third-party payment, and may favorably influence liability insurance premiums.

Major Initiatives

The Joint Commission works to improve the quality of health care through such projects as the ORYX initiative, which is establishing performance measurement requirements and supporting quality improvement efforts within accredited organization. The ultimate objective is to integrate outcomes and other performance measurement data into the accreditation process.

Consumers can gain information on JCAHO-accredited health care organizations on-line through Quality Check™, which is accessible through the Joint Commission's Web site at www.jcaho.org. Performance reports, providing more detailed information about each accredited institution, are also available through Quality Check™.

Origins/Governance

The Joint Commission was founded in 1951. Its governing Board of Commissioners consists of 28 individuals with experience that is broadly representative of the health care field. The board includes practicing physicians, health care executives, and public members whose expertise includes bioethics, nursing, labor relations, business, insurance, education, and quality improvement, among others. The board's direct link to the current health care environment enables it to guide the Joint Commission in developing state-of-the-art evaluation services.

JCAHO
One Renaissance Blvd
Oakbrook Terrace, IL 60181
630 792-5000   630 792-5005 Fax
www.jcaho.org

National Association Medical Staff Services

Formed in 1978, the National Association Medical Staff Services (NAMSS) is an international association that provides professional education resources to individuals in the areas of health care credentialing, clinical privileging, practitioner/provider organizations, and regulatory compliance. Its mission is to protect and promote high-quality health care for the public by helping its members understand and succeed in the changing organizational structures of the health care industry. It also develops, administers, and promotes certification programs that measure knowledge of current industry standards and practices.

For more information, contact:

National Association Medical Staff Services
8317 Cross Park Dr/#150
Austin, TX 78754
512 454-7928
512 381-6036 Fax
www.namss.org

National Committee for Quality Assurance

The National Committee for Quality Assurance (NCQA) is a private, not-for-profit organization that assesses and reports on the quality of managed care plans, providing a basis for purchasers and consumers of managed health care to distinguish among plans. The efforts of the NCQA are organized around accreditation and performance measurement.

Origins and Scope

The NCQA began accrediting managed care organizations (MCOs) in 1991 in response to the need for standardized, objective information about the quality of these organizations. Since then, its has expanded the range of organizations that it accredits or certifies to include managed behavioral health care organizations, credentials verification organizations, and physician organizations. More than 75% of all Americans covered by HMOs are in HMOs that have been reviewed by the NCQA.

Accreditation

More than half the HMOs in the nation are currently involved in the NCQA accreditation process. Organizations seeking NCQA accreditation must undergo a survey and meet certain standards designed to evaluate the health plan's clinical and administrative systems, including efforts to continuously improve the quality of care and service it delivers.

During an accreditation survey, plans are reviewed against more than 50 standards, which fall into six categories:

- Quality improvement (40% of a plan's score)
- Physician credentials (20%)
- Members' rights and responsibilities (10%)
- Preventive health services (15%)
- Utilization management (10%)
- Medical records (5%)

NCQA accreditation surveys are conducted by teams of physicians and managed care experts. A national oversight committee of physicians analyzes the team's findings and assigns one of four possible accreditation levels (full, 1-year, provisional, or denial) based on the plan's level of compliance with NCQA standards.

Performance Measurement

HEDIS
In addition to examining a health plan's structures and systems through accreditation, the NCQA looks at the results or outcomes the plan actually achieves. It manages the principal performance measurement tool for managed care, the Health Plan Employer Data and Information Set (HEDIS), a set of 71 standardized measures used to evaluate and compare health plans.

Work related to HEDIS has led to projects in distributing performance data, ensuring data accuracy, and making sure the performance data are useful to help guide choice. The NCQA's work in the area of performance measurement focuses on four key areas: HEDIS; NCQA's Quality Compass (a national database of HEDIS data and accreditation information); audit procedures; and consumer research.

Performance Measurement Coordinating Council
To bring consistency to their independent assessment initiatives, NCQA, the Joint Commission on Accreditation of Healthcare Organizations, and the American Medical Accreditation Program have formed the Performance Measurement Coordinating Council, through which they will collaborate to develop and implement coherent and efficient performance measures in health care.

For more information, contact:

National Committee for Quality Assurance
2000 L St NW/Ste 500
Washington, DC 20036
202 955-3500
202 955-3599 Fax
www.ncqa.org

Appendixes

Appendix A

Boards of Medical Examiners in the United States and Possessions

Larry Dixon, Executive Director
Alabama Board of Medical Examiners
PO Box 946
848 Washington Ave
Montgomery, AL 36101-0946
334 242-4116
334 242-4155 Fax
www.bmedixon.home.mindspring.com

Leslie Abel, Executive Administrator
Alaska State Medical Board
Division of Occupational Licensing
3601 C St, Ste 722
Anchorage, AK 99503-5986
907 269-8160
907 269-8156 Fax
E-mail: Leslie_Abel@commerce.state.ak.us
www.commerce.state.ak.us/occ

Claudia Foutz, Executive Director
Arizona Board of Medical Examiners
9545 E Doubletree Ranch Rd
Scottsdale, AZ 85258
480 551-2700
480 551-2704 Fax
www.docboard.org/bomex

Peggy Pryor Cryer, Executive Secretary
Arkansas State Medical Board
2100 Riverfront Dr, Ste 200
Little Rock, AR 72202-1793
501 296-1802
501 296-1805 Fax
E-mail: asmb@mail.state.ar.us

Ronald Joseph, Executive Director
Medical Board of California
1426 Howe Ave, Ste 56
Sacramento, CA 95825-3236
916 263-2389
916 263-2387 Fax
www.medbd.ca.gov or www.docboard.org

Susan Miller, Program Administrator
Colorado Board of Medical Examiners
1560 Broadway, Ste 1300
Denver, CO 80202-5140
303 894-7690
303 894-7692 Fax
E-mail: susan.miller@dora.state.co.us
www.dora.state.co.us/medical

Jennifer Filipone, Health Program Supervisor
State of Connecticut, Department of Public Health
Physician Licensure Unit
PO Box 340308, 410 Capital Ave, MS #12APP
Hartford, CT 06134-0308
860 509-7563
860 509-8457 Fax
www.state.ct.us/dph/

Douglas Reed, Executive Director
Delaware Board of Medical Practice
861 Silver Lake Blvd, Ste 203
Dover, DE 19903
302 739-4522 x229
302 739-2711 Fax
E-mail: dreed@state.de.us

Robert B Vowels, MD, Acting Executive Director
District of Columbia Board of Medicine
825 North Capitol St NE, Rm 2224
Washington, DC 20002
202 224-4777
202 442-9431 Fax

Tanya Williams, Executive Director
Florida Board of Medicine
Bin # C03
4052 Bald Cypress Way
Tallahassee, FL 32399-1753
850 245-4131
850 922-3040 Fax
www.doh.state.fl.us

Karen Mason, Executive Director
Georgia Composite State Board of Medical Examiners
2 Peachtree Street, 6th Floor
Atlanta, GA 30303
404 656-3913
404 656-9723 Fax
www.sos.state.ga.us/ebd-medical

Teofilia P Cruz, RN MS, Executive Director
Guam Board of Medical Examiners
PO Box 2816
1304 E Sunset Blvd
Agana, GU 96910-2816
671 475-0251 or 0252
671 477-4733 Fax
E-mail: tcruz@ncsbn.org

Constance Cabral-Makanani, Executive Director
Hawaii Board of Medical Examiners
1010 Richards St
Honolulu, HI 96813
808 586-2708
808 586-2874 Fax

Darleene Thorsted, Executive Director
Idaho State Board of Medicine
PO Box 83720
Boise, ID 83720-0058
208 327-7000
208 327-7005 Fax
E-mail: tsolt@bom.state.id.us

Alicia Purchase, Manager, Medical Unit
Illinois Board of Medical Examiners
Department of Professional Regulation
320 W Washington, 3rd Fl, Med-1
Springfield, IL 62786
217 782-8556
217 524-2169 Fax
www.state.il.us/dpr

Laura Langford, RN, Executive Director
Indiana Health Professions Bureau
402 W Washington St, Rm 041
Indianapolis, IN 46204
317 232-2960
317 233-4236 Fax
www.ai.org/hpb

Ann Mowery, PhD, Executive Director
Iowa Board of Medical Examiners
Suite C, 400 SW 8th Street
Des Moines, IA 50309-4686
515 281-5171
515 242-5908 Fax
E-mail: amowery@bon.state.ia.us
www.docboard.org

Lawrence Buening, Executive Director
Kansas Board of Healing Arts
235 SW Topeka Blvd
Topeka, KS 66603-3068
785 296-7413
785 296-8052 Fax
www.ink.org/public/boha or www.docboard.org/aim.htm

C Schmidt, Executive Director
Kentucky Board of Medical Licensure
310 Whittington Pkwy, Ste 1B
Louisville, KY 40222
502 429-8046
502 429-9923 Fax

Virginia Benoist, Executive Director
Louisiana State Board of Medical Examiners
PO Box 30250
630 Camp St
New Orleans, LA 70130-0250
504 524-6763
504 568-8893 Fax
www.lsbme.org

Randal Manning, Executive Director
Maine Board of Licensure in Medicine
Two Bangor St
137 State House Station
Augusta, ME 04333
207 287-3601
207 287-6590 Fax
www.docboard.org/aim.htm

J Compton, Executive Director
Maryland Board of Physician Quality Assurance
PO Box 2571
4201 Patterson Ave, 3rd Fl
Baltimore, MD 21215-0095
410 764-4777
410 358-2252 Fax
E-mail: bpqa@erols.com
www.docboard.org/aim.htm

Nancy Achin Sullivan
Massachusetts Board of Registration in Medicine
10 West St, 3rd Fl
Boston, MA 02111
617 727-3086
617 451-9568 Fax
www.docboard.org/aim.htm

Bureau of Health Services
Michigan Board of Medicine
611 W Ottawa St
Lansing, MI 48933
517 373-6873
517 241-3082 Fax
www.cis.state.mi.us/bhser

Robert Leach, JD, Executive Director
Minnesota Board of Medical Practice
University Park Plaza
2829 University Ave SE, Ste 400
Minneapolis, MN 55414-3246
612 617-2130
612 617-2166 Fax
www.bmp.state.mn.us or www.docboard.org/aim.htm

W Joseph Burnett, MD, Director
Mississippi State Board of Medical Licensure
1867 Crane Ridge Dr, Ste 200B
Jackson, MS 39216
601 987-3079
601 987-4159 Fax
E-mail: mboard@msbml.state.ms.us
www.msbml.state.ms.us

Tina Steinman, Executive Director
Missouri State Board of Registration for the Healing Arts
Division of Professional Regulation
PO Box 4, 3605 Missouri Blvd
Jefferson City, MO 65102-0004
573 751-0098
573 751-3166 Fax
www.ecodev.state.mo.us/pr/healarts

Patricia England, JD, Executive Secretary
Montana Board of Medical Examiners
PO Box 200513
111 N Jackson
Helena, MT 59620-0513
406 444-1988
406 444-9396 Fax

Katherine Brown, Team Leader
Nebraska Health and Human Services System
Dept of Regulation and Licensure, Credentialing Div
301 Centennial Mall South, PO Box 94986
Lincoln, NE 68509-4986
402 471-2118
402 471-3577 Fax
E-mail: vicki.bumgarner@hhss.state.ne.us
www.hhs.state.ne.us/lis/lis.asp

Larry Lessly, JD, Executive Director
Nevada State Board of Medical Examiners
PO Box 7238
1105 Terminal Way, Ste 301
Reno, NV 89502
775 688-2559
775 688-2321 Fax
E-mail: nsbme@govmail.state.nv.us
www.state.nv.us/medical

Penny Taylor, Acting Administrator
New Hampshire Board of Medicine
2 Industrial Park Dr, Ste 8
Concord, NH 03301-8520
603 271-1205
603 271-6702 Fax
www.state.nh.us/medicine

William Roeder, Executive Director
New Jersey State Board of Medical Examiners
PO Box 183
140 E Front Street, 2nd Fl
Trenton, NJ 08645-0183
609 826-7100
609 777-0956 Fax
www.state.nj.us/lps/ca/bme

Kristen Hedrick, MPH, Executive Director
New Mexico Board of Medical Examiners
Lamy Bldg, 2nd Fl
491 Old Santa Fe Trail
Santa Fe, NM 87501
505 827-7363
505 827-7377 Fax

Thomas Monahan, Executive Secretary
New York State Education Department
Cultural Education Center, Rm 3023
Empire State Plaza
Albany, NY 12230
518 474-3841
518 486-4846 Fax
E-mail: medbd@mail.nysed.gov
www.op.nysed.gov

Andy Watry, Executive Director
North Carolina Medical Board
1201 Front St
PO Box 20007
Raleigh, NC 27609
919 326-1100 ext 221
919 326-1130 or Fax 326-1131
www.docboard.org/nc/nc_home.htm

Rolf Sletten, JD, Executive Secretary and Treasurer
North Dakota Board of Medical Examiners
418 E Broadway Ave, Ste 12
Bismarck, ND 58501
701 328-6500
701 328-6505 Fax
E-mail: bomex@tic.bisman.com
www.ndbomex.com

Thomas Dilling, Executive Director
State Medical Board of Ohio
77 S High St, 17th Fl
Columbus, OH 43215
614 466-3934
614 728-5946 Fax
E-mail: thomas.dilling@med.state.oh.us
www.state.oh.us/med

Lyle Kelsey, Executive Director
Oklahoma Board of Medical Licensure and Supervision
PO Box 18256
Oklahoma City, OK 73154-0256
405 848-6841
405 848-8240 Fax
E-mail: executive@osbmls.state.ok.us
www.osbmls.state.ok.us

Kathleen Haley, JD, Executive Director
Oregon Board of Medical Examiners
620 Crown Plaza
1500 SW First Ave
Portland, OR 97201-5826
503 229-5770
503 229-6543 Fax

Cindy Warner, Administrative Officer
Pennsylvania State Board of Medicine
PO Box 2649, 116 Pine St
Harrisburg, PA 17101
717 787-2381
717 787-7769 Fax

Ivonne Fernandez Colon, Executive Director
Puerto Rico Board of Medical Examiners
Department of Health
PO Box 13969
San Juan, PR 00908
787 782-8989
787 782-8733 Fax

Milton Hamolsky, MD, Chief Administrative Officer
Rhode Island Board of Medical Licensure and Discipline
Joseph E Cannon Bldg, Rm 205
Three Capitol Hill
Providence, RI 02908-5097
401 222-3855
401 222-2158 Fax
www.docboard.org/ri/main.htm

John D. Volmer, Board Administrator
South Carolina Department of Labor, Licensing and Regulation
PO Box 11289
110 Centerview Dr, Ste 202
Columbia, SC 29211-1289
803-896-4500
803 896-4515 Fax
E-mail: medboard@mail.llr.state.sc.us
www.llr.state.sc.us/me.htm

Robert Johnson, Executive Secretary
South Dakota State Board of Medical & Osteopathic Examiners
1323 S Minnesota Ave
Sioux Falls, SD 57105
605 334-8343
605 336-0270 Fax

Yarnell Beatty, Executive Director
Tennessee Department of Health
First Floor, Cordell Hull Bldg
426 Fifth Ave N
Nashville, TN 37247-1010
615 532-4384
615 253-4484 Fax
www.state.tn.us/health

Frank Langley, MD JD, Executive Director
Texas State Board of Medical Examiners
PO Box 2018
Austin, TX 78768-2018
512 305-7010
512 305-7006 Fax
www.tsbme.state.tx.us or www.docboard.org/aim.htm

Peter Duke, Bureau Manager
State of Utah Department of Commerce
Division of Occupational & Professional Licensing
PO Box 146741, 160 East 300 South
Salt Lake City, UT 84114-6741
801 530-6628
801 530-6511 Fax
www.commerce.state.ut.us

Barbara Neuman, JD, Executive Director
Vermont Board of Medical Practice
109 State St
Montpelier, VT 05609-1106
802 828-2673
802 828-5450 Fax
www.sec.state.vt.us or www.docboard.org/aim.htm

Lydia Scott, Executive Assistant
Virgin Islands Board of Medical Examiners
Office of the Commissioner, Department of Health
48 Sugar Estate
St Thomas, VI 00802
340 774-0117
340 777-4001 Fax

William Harp, MD, Executive Director
Virginia Board of Medicine
6606 W Broad St, 4th Fl
Richmond, VA 23230-1717
804 662-9960
804 662-9517 Fax
E-mail: medbd@dhp.state.va.us
www.dhp.state.va.us

Bonnie King, Executive Director
Washington State Department of Public Health
Medical Quality Assurance Commission
PO Box 47866, 1300 SE Quince St
Olympia, WA 98504-7866
360 236-4789
360 586-8480 Fax
E-mail: blk0303@hub.doh.wa.gov
www.doh.wa.gov

Ronald Walton, Executive Director
West Virginia Board of Medicine
101 Dee Dr
Charleston, WV 25311
304 558-2921
304 558-2084 Fax

Patrick Braatz, Bureau Director
State of Wisconsin Medical Examining Board
Bureau of Health Professions, Dept of Regulation & Licensing
PO Box 8935, 1400 E Washington Ave
Madison, WI 53708-8935
608 266-0483
608 267-1803 Fax

Carole Shotwell, JD, Executive Secretary
Wyoming Board of Medicine
Colony Bldg, 2nd Fl
211 W 19th St
Cheyenne, WY 82002
307 778-7053
307 778-2069 Fax
E-mail: wyobom@aol.com

Appendix B
Boards of Osteopathic Medical Examiners in the United States and Possessions

Ann Marie Berger, Executive Secretary
Arizona Board of Osteopathic Examiners in Medicine and Surgery
9535 E Doubletree Ranch Rd
Scottsdale, AZ 85258
480 657-7703   480 657-7715 Fax

Linda Bergmann, Executive Director
Osteopathic Medical Board of California
2720 Gateway Oaks Dr, Ste 350
Sacramento, CA 95833-3500
916 263-3100   916 263-3117 Fax
E-mail: ombc@pacbell.net

Tonya Williams, Executive Director
Florida Board of Osteopathic Medicine
Bin C03
4052 Bald Cypress Way
Tallahassee, FL 32399-1753
850 488-0595   850 922-3040 Fax

Susan Strout, Executive Secretary
Maine Board of Osteopathic Licensure
142 State House Station
Augusta, ME 04333
207 287-2480   207 287-2480 Fax

Carol Engle, Director of Licensing
Michigan Board of Osteopathic Medicine and Surgery
611 W Ottawa St
Lansing, MI 48933
517 335-7222   517 335-4478 Fax

Larry Tarno, DO, Executive Director
Nevada State Board of Osteopathic Medicine
2950 E Flamingo Rd, Ste E3
Las Vegas, NV 89121-5208
702 732-2147   702 732-2079 Fax

Elizabeth Montoya, Executive Director
New Mexico Board of Osteopathic Medical Examiners
PO Box 25101
725 St Michaels Dr
Santa Fe, NM 87504
505 476-7120   505 476-7095 Fax

Gary Clark, Executive Director
Oklahoma Board of Osteopathic Examiners
4848 N Lincoln Blvd, Ste 100
Oklahoma City, OK 73105-3321
405 528-8625   405 557-0653 Fax

Gina Bittner, Administrative Assistant
Pennsyslvania State Board of Osteopathic Medicine
PO Box 2649
116 Pine St
Harrisburg, PA 17101
717 783-4858   717 787-7769 Fax

Yarnell Beatty, Director
Tennessee State Board of Osteopathic Examiners
First Floor, Cordell Hull Bldg
426 Fifth Ave N
Nashville, TN 37247-1010
615 532-5080   615 532-5164 Fax

Peggy Atkins, Staff Secretary
Vermont Board of Osteopathic Physicians and Surgeons
Vermont Section of State Office
Office of Professional Regulations
109 State St
Montpelier, VT 05602-1106
802 828-2373   802 828-2465 Fax
E-mail: patkins@sec.state.vt.us

Arlene Robertson, Program Manager
Washington Board of Osteopathic Medicine and Surgery
Department of Health
PO Box 47870
Olympia, WA 98504-7870
360 236-4944   360 586-0745 Fax
E-mail: ean@303@hub.doh.wa.gov

Joseph Schreiber, DO, Secretary
West Virginia Board of Osteopathy
334 Penco Rd
Weirton, WV 26062
304 723-4638   304 293-6685 Fax

Appendix C

Member Boards of the Federation of Medical Licensing Authorities of Canada

Sylvia Smith, Executive Secretary
Federation of Medical Licensing Authorities of Canada
2283 St Laurent Blvd, PO Box 8234
Ottawa, ON K1G 3H7
613 738-0372   613 738-8977 Fax

L R Ohlhauser, MD, Registrar
College of Physicians and Surgeons of Alberta
900 Manulife Place, 10180-101 St
Edmonton, AB T5J 4P8
780 423-4764   780 420-0651 Fax
http://www.cpsa.ab.ca

T F Handley, MD, Registrar
College of Physicians & Surgeons of British Columbia
1807 W 10th Ave
Vancouver, BC V6J 2A9
604 733-7758   604 733-3503 Fax

W Pope, MD, Registrar
College of Physicians and Surgeons of Manitoba
494 St James St
Winnipeg, MB R3G 3J4
204 774-4344   204 774-0750 Fax
http://www.umanitoba.ca/colleges/cps

E Schollenberg, MD, Registrar
College of Physicians and Surgeons of New Brunswick
One Hampton Rd, Ste 300
Rothesay, NB E2E 5K8
506 849-5050   506 849-5069 Fax
http://www.cpsnb.org

R W Young, MD, Registrar
Newfoundland Medical Board
139 Water St
St John's, NF A1C 1B2
709 726-8546   709 726-4725 Fax

C Little, MD, Registrar
College of Physicians and Surgeons of Nova Scotia
200-1559 Brunswick St, Sentry Pl
Halifax, NS B3J 2E1
902 422-5823   902 422-5035 Fax
http://www.cpsns.ns.ca

Jeannette Hall, Registrar, Professional Licensing
Government of the Northwest Territories
Department of Health and Social Service
Centre Square Tower, 8th Fl, PO Box 1320
Yellowknife, NWT X1A 2L9
867 920-8058   867 873-0281 Fax

J Bonn, MD, Registrar
College of Physicians and Surgeons of Ontario
80 College St
Toronto, ON M5G 2E2
416 967-2600   416 961-3330 Fax
http://www.cpso.on.ca

C Moyse, MD, Registrar
College of Physicians and Surgeons of Prince Edward Island
199 Grafton St
Charlottetown, PEI C1A 1L2
902 566-3861   902 566-3861 Fax

J Lescop, MD, Secrétaire-générale
College des médecins du Québec
2170 boul René Lévésque ouest
Montréal, PQ H3H 2T8
514 933-4441   514 933-3112 Fax
http://www.cmg.org

D A Kendel, MD, Registrar
College of Physicians and Surgeons of Saskatchewan
211 4th Ave S
Saskatoon, SK S7K 1N1
306 244-7355   306 244-0090 Fax

Elsie Bagan, Registrar, Medical Practitioners
Department of Consumer and Corporate Affairs
Government of the Yukon
PO Box 2703
Whitehorse, YT Y1A 2C6
867 667-5257   867 667-3609 Fax

Appendix D

Glossary of Medical Licensure Terms and List of Common Abbreviations

Common Abbreviations

ABMS	American Board of Medical Specialties
ACGME	Accreditation Council for Graduate Medical Education
AMAP	American Medical Accreditation Program
AMA PRA	American Medical Association Physician's Recognition Award
AOA	American Osteopathic Association
CME	Continuing medical education
COMLEX	Comprehensive Osteopathic Medical Licensing Examination
ECFMG	Educational Commission for Foreign Medical Graduates
FLEX	Federation Licensing Examination
FSMB	Federation of State Medical Boards
FWA	Federation Licensing Examination (FLEX) Weighted Average
GMC	Graduate Medical Council (United Kingdom)
GME	Graduate medical education
IMG	International medical graduate
JCAHO	Joint Commission on Accreditation of Healthcare Organizations
LCME	Liaison Committee on Medical Education
LMCC	Licentiate of the Medical Council of Canada
NAMSS	National Association Medical Staff Services
NBME	National Board of Medical Examiners
NBOME	National Board of Osteopathic Medical Examiners
NCQA	National Committee for Quality Assurance
PRA	American Medical Association Physician's Recognition Award
SBE	State board examination
SPEX	Special Purpose Examination
USMLE	United States Medical Licensing Examination
VQE	Visa Qualifying Examination
WHO	World Health Organization

Definitions

Accreditation Council for Graduate Medical Education (ACGME)

An accrediting agency composed of representatives from five national associations interested in graduate medical education (each of which appoints four directors), in addition to a federal government representative, three public directors chosen by the ACGME, and a resident physician director. The chair of the Residency Review Committee Council, an ACGME advisory body, participates in ACGME meetings in a voting capacity. The ACGME, through its 27 review committees (26 Residency Review Committees, or RRCs, and the Transitional Year Review Committee), accredits graduate medical education programs.

American Board of Medical Specialties (ABMS)

A nonprofit organization of 24 approved medical specialty boards. Its mission is to maintain and improve the quality of medical care by helping its member boards develop and use professional and educational standards for the evaluation and certification of physician specialists. The certification of physicians provides assurance to the public that a physician specialist certified by an ABMS member board has successfully completed an approved educational program and an evaluation process that assesses the knowledge, skills, and experience required to provide quality patient care in that specialty. Medical specialty board certification is an additional process to receiving a medical degree, completing residency training, and receiving a license to practice medicine.

Certification

A voluntary process intended to assure the public that a certified medical specialist has successfully completed an approved educational program and an evaluation including an examination process designed to assess the knowledge, experience, and skills requisite to the provision of high-quality patient care in that specialty.

Clerkship

Clinical education provided to medical students.

Educational Commission for Foreign Medical Graduates (ECFMG)

A nonprofit organization that assesses the readiness of graduates of foreign medical schools to enter residency programs in the United States accredited by the Accreditation Council for Graduate Medical Education (ACGME).

ECFMG certification provides assurance to directors of ACGME-accredited residency programs, and to the people of the United States, that graduates of foreign medical schools have met minimum standards of eligibility required to enter such programs. This certification does not guarantee that such graduates will be accepted into these programs in the United States, since the number of applicants frequently exceeds the number of positions available.

ECFMG certification is also a prerequisite required by most states for licensure to practice medicine in the United States and is one of the eligibility requirements to take Step 3 of the United States Medical Licensing Examination (USMLE).

ECFMG number

The number assigned by the Educational Commission for Foreign Medical Graduates (ECFMG) to each international medical graduate (IMG) who applies for certification from ECFMG. Almost all graduates of foreign medical schools must have an ECFMG certificate to participate in graduate medical education in the US.

Fellow

An individual undertaking post-residency training in a field of research or clinical practice that is not accredited by the Accreditation Council for Graduate Medical Education (ACGME). In some instances, the term "fellow" is used to designate resident physicians in subspecialty GME programs, but both the AMA and ACGME prefer the use of "resident" or "resident physician" to designate individuals in all ACGME-accredited programs. *Also see "Resident or resident physician."*

Fifth Pathway

One of several ways that individuals who obtain their undergraduate medical education abroad can enter GME in the United States. The Fifth Pathway is a period of supervised clinical training for students who obtained their premedical education in the United States, received undergraduate medical education abroad, and passed Step 1 of the United States Medical Licensing Examination. After these students successfully complete a year of clinical training sponsored by US medical school accredited by the Liaison Committee on Medical Education (LCME) and pass USMLE Step 2, they receive a Fifth Pathway certificate and become eligible for an ACGME-accredited residency as an international medical graduate. Currently, New York Medical College in Valhalla, New York is the only medical school that offers the Fifth Pathway.

Federation Licensing Examination (FLEX)

Originally introduced in 1968 and subsequently enhanced and modified in 1985, this examination was administered for the last time in December 1993. In 1994, the United States Medical Licensing Examination (USMLE) was fully implemented. Some candidates for licensure may have a combination of scores from FLEX and USMLE. *Also see "United States Medical Licensing Examination."*

Federation of State Medical Boards (FSMB)

A nonprofit organization whose membership comprises the 69 medical licensing boards of all US states, the District of Columbia, Guam, Puerto Rico, and the Virgin Islands, as well as most of the separate osteopathic licensing boards in the United States. Its primary responsibility is to protect the public through the regulation of physicians and other health care providers. It serves as a liaison, advocate, and information source to the public, health care organizations, and state, national, and international authorities. The FSMB promotes high standards for physician licensure and practice and assists and supports state medical boards collectively and individually in the regulation of medical practice and in their role of public protection.

FLEX Weighted Average (FWA)

All states currently require a minimum passing score of 75 on each component of the post-1985 two-part FLEX; the resulting number composes the Federation Licensing Examination (FLEX) Weighted Average.

International medical graduate (IMG)

A graduate of a medical school not accredited by the Liaison Committee on Medical Education (LCME). Formerly referred to as "foreign medical graduate" (FMG).

Initial license

The first ever full and unrestricted license a physician receives in his/her medical career. Some medical boards interpret "initial license" as a physician's first license in their particular states (although the physician could already have been licensed in other states). This publication does not use the term in this sense.

Licensure

The process by which a state or jurisdiction of the United States admits physicians to the practice of medicine. Licensure ensures that practicing physicians have appropriate education and training and that they abide by recognized standards of professional conduct while serving their patients. Candidates for first licensure must complete a rigorous examination designed to assess a physician's ability to apply knowledge, concepts, and principles that are important in health and disease and that constitute the basis of safe and effective patient care. All applicants must submit proof of medical education and training and provide details about their work history. Finally, applicants must reveal information regarding past medical history (including the use of habit-forming drugs and emotional or mental illness), arrests, and convictions. *Also see "Limited license" and "Reregistration."*

Limited license

Issued by state medical boards to resident physicians in graduate medical education (GME) programs within their jurisdictions. Physicians do not receive a full and unrestricted license until completion of GME and fulfillment of other licensure requirements in a given jurisdiction.

Locum tenens

This Latin term (locum "place," tenens "to hold") describes a person taking another's place for the time being. In medicine, for example, the American Medical Association's Project USA provides short-term replacements for US Public Health Service physicians in rural locations, allowing them to take a vacation or fulfill continuing medical education requirements (see "Project USA," p. 92).

Medical Practice Act

A statute of a US state or jurisdiction that outlines the practice of medicine and the responsibility of the medical board to regulate that practice. The primary responsibility and obligation of a state medical board is to protect the public through proper licensing and regulation of physicians and, in some jurisdictions, other health care professionals. *Also see "Unprofessional conduct."*

National Board of Medical Examiners (NBME)

A nonprofit, independent organization that prepares and administers medical qualifying examinations, either independently or jointly with other organizations. Legal agencies governing the practice of medicine within each US state or jurisdiction may grant a license without further examination for those physicians who have successfully completed such examinations and met other requirements.

Certification by the NBME can be used as an avenue to licensure in the United States for those certified as diplomates prior to implementation of the United State Medical Licensing Examination (USMLE) and for examinees taking a combination of NBME and/or USMLE examinations who passed at least one part or step before December 31, 1994. The last regular administration of Part I occurred in 1991, Part II in April 1992, and Part III in May 1994.

Currently, the NBME administers USMLE Steps 1 and 2 to students and graduates of US and Canadian medical schools accredited by the Liaison Committee on Medical Education or the American Osteopathic Association.

Reregistration

After physicians are licensed in a state or jurisdiction, they must reregister periodically to continue their active status. During this reregistration process, physicians are required to demonstrate that they have maintained acceptable standards of ethics and medical practice and have not engaged in improper conduct. In some states, physicians must also show that they have participated in a program of continuing medical education.

Resident or resident physician

Any individual at any level in an ACGME-accredited GME program, including subspecialty programs. Local usage might refer to these individuals as interns, house officers, house staff, trainees, fellows, or junior faculty. *Also see "Fellow."*

Special Purpose Examination (SPEX)

This 1-day, computer-administered examination, with approximately 420 multiple-choice questions, assesses primary care medical knowledge and skills. It does not include questions specific to a particular specialty or subspecialty. The SPEX is used to assess physicians who have held a valid, unrestricted license in a US or Canadian jurisdiction who are:

- required by the state medical board to demonstrate current medical knowledge,
- seeking endorsement licensure some years beyond initial examination, or
- seeking license reinstatement after a period of professional inactivity.

Physicians holding a valid, unrestricted license may also apply for SPEX, independent of any request or approval from a medical licensing board.

Telemedicine

Telemedicine is the delivery of health care services via electronic means from a health care provider in one location to a patient in another. Applications that fall under this definition include the transfer of medical images, such as pathology slides or radiographs, interactive video consultations between patient and provider or between primary care and specialty care physicians, and mental health consultations (see Table 15 for more information).

Unprofessional conduct

Although laws vary from one jurisdiction to the next, the Medical Practice Acts in force in most US jurisdictions would define unprofessional conduct as including:

- physical abuse of a patient
- inadequate recordkeeping
- not recognizing or acting on common symptoms
- prescribing drugs in excessive amounts or without legitimate reason
- impaired ability to practice due to addiction or physical or mental illness
- failing to meet continuing medical education requirements
- performing duties beyond the scope of a license
- dishonesty
- conviction of a felony
- the practice of medicine to an unlicensed individual

Unprofessional conduct would not include minor disagreements or poor customer service.

United States Medical Licensing Examination (USMLE)

This 3-step examination for US medical licensure provides a common evaluation system for applicants. The USMLE program is governed by a composite committee of representatives from the Federation of State Medical Boards (FSMB), the National Board of Medical Examiners (NBME), the Educational Commission for Foreign Medical Graduates (ECFMG), and the public.

Results of the USMLE are reported to state medical boards for use in granting the initial license to practice medicine. Each medical licensing authority requires, as part of its licensing processes, successful completion of an examination or other certification demonstrating qualification for licensure.

The USMLE replaced FLEX and the certifying examination of the NBME, as well as the Foreign Medical Graduate Examination in the Medical Sciences (FMGEMS), which was formerly used by the ECFMG for certification purposes. Steps 1 and 2 of the USMLE are used as the examination for ECFMG certification. These two steps are also used for promotion and graduation in some US medical schools.